8/14/21

DARK MATTERS - DARK SECRETS

To My Sis

Des

T. Owens Moore, Ph.D.

Thank you for the support and may this reading be an "endarkening" experience!

With Essence,

Dr. T.O. Moore

AF837258

Zamani Press
P.O. Box 667
Redan, GA 30074

Copyright © 2002 T. Owens Moore, Ph.D.

Published by:
Zamani Press
P.O. Box 667
Redan, GA 30074
Website: http://www.zamanipress.com
E-mail: tmoore@zamanipress.com

All rights reserved. No part of this book may be reproduced in any form without written permission from the Publishers, except by a reviewer who may quote brief passages in a review to be printed in a newspaper or magazine.

First published 2002
Second printing 2005

ISBN 1-884897-02-9 (pbk.)

1. Melanin. 2. Black Studies. 3. Psychology. 4. Science. 5. Drug Addiction.

Cover Illustration: King Akhenaten and Queen Nerfertiti and their children are relaxing in the midst of almighty RA (i.e., the sun). After years of thought, Akhenaten determined that only the solar gods were worthy of veneration, and that their worship must take the place of the God Amen. Akhenaten adopted the sun disk (ATEN) as his symbol of God. Note how Ancient Africans represented ankhs at the ends of the rays to symbolize the breadth of life to the nostrils.

DEDICATION

To my daughter Jemila Njeri:
Your inquisitive mind provides the
inspiration for these endarkening words.

Contents

ACKNOWLEDGMENTS

In the process of preparing a follow up text to the 1995 edition of *The Science of Melanin*, my colleague and comrade (Dr. Jelani Madaraka) from Zamani Press suggested that I had a wealth of information that could be divided into more than one book. Your suggestion to split my discourse on melanin into separate volumes was very informative. The option was considered, however, it was more feasible to present one book for this second treatise on melanin. I followed the recommendation to appropriately decipher the information for the interested reader, and I am grateful for your assistance in the preparation of this book. Dr. Madaraka, may you continue to be blessed with intellectual insight, and long live Zamani Press.

In proof reading the initial manuscript, I thank Dr. Bruce Bynum and Frederick Scott for taking your valuable time to help me formulate a plan for this text. Dr. Russell Kelley, Bruce Muhammad and Nkosua Reedy, your support and helpful comments were also appreciated.

I have asked myself, "How do you write acknowledgments when there are so many people who have contributed to your spiritual awareness and mental consciousness?" The Association of Black Psychologists and the many African-centered scholars I have learned from are integral to my success. Leaders in the field of African-centered Psychology such as Drs. Naim Akbar, Asa Hilliard, Kobi Kambon, Linda James-Myers, Wade Nobles, Kathleen Burlew and Halford Fairchild, just to name a few, have quietly shown to me what it means to lead in an African-centered direction. Without the vision of the founders, the leaders and the work force of the Association of Black Psychologists, there would be minimal interest in concepts related to "Blackness." I acknowledge the ABPsi for spiritual rejuvenation and the Howard University Psychology Faculty who introduced me to provocative information about people of African descent.

In addition, my students are a major source of my strength. They have kept me committed to the task of providing positive information about people of African descent. As the students yearn for information, we as African-centered scholars are responsible for setting the mental sails in the right direction. For who else can be committed to molding the minds of our youth and creating a ocean of possibility for them except for those who are willing to explore unchartered territory. The students are too numerous to mention, but I thank all of you for wanting to know more about yourself. In discovering yourself, you teach the world to become a better place and to reach new horizons.

In sum, the excitement for the preparation of this book is solely due to the people who have generated an interest in the topic. I was often asked when is the next book coming and I could never provide an adequate response. Although long overdue, I have finally completed the follow up text to *The Science of Melanin.* I acknowledge each and every person in the community and the research field who has been endarkened by the topic and who has desired to read more. Last, but not least, I would like to thank my wife Teresa and three children (Tyehimba, Jabari and Jemila) for your moral support. Many thanks to my mother Esther Moore for spiritual support. Finally, I acknowledge all of my family members and dear friends because I am comforted to know that you will always believe in me.

PREFACE

A scientific discussion of the topic of melanin research can be both intriguing and complex. For example, speculating on the role of melanin in human behavior is intriguing, but it is a challenge to decipher the scientific jargon that describes melanin functioning. Without a thorough understanding of some basic concepts, it may be difficult to understand the reason why melanin is an important biological entity. *The Science of Melanin: Dispelling the Myths* was written in 1995 as a primer to understand the complex area of melanin research. As a continuing exploration, *Dark Matters* was written to discuss the physiological effects of melanin in the skin and in the central nervous system. *Dark Secrets* was written to discuss how the biological properties of melanin can affect a person's susceptibility to drug abuse and addiction. *The Science of Melanin: Dispelling Myths* has been reprinted and published by another company. Although the content is the same, the subtitle has been changed to *Exposing the Truth*. In sum, the first and second book should provide the reader with a comprehensive analysis of melanin research from an African-centered perspective.

Considering the numerous scientific studies on melanin, there are not many African-centered approaches to the area of melanin research (King, 1990, 1994; Barnes, 1988, 1993; Pookrum, 1993; Welsing, 1991; Andrews, 1989; Amen, 1993), so this text will be an added source of information. Many scholars have discussed melanin in lectures as well as cited melanin concepts in their research. Most recently, ideas centered on melanin research have been introduced in major texts in the area of African/Black Psychology (Kambon, 1998) and as an underlying theme in African-centered concepts in psychology (Bynum, 1999).

In Part One, *Dark Matters*, we speculate on the role of melanin outside of its effects on skin pigmentation. From a sociopolitical perspective, dark skin has been a reason to subjugate a whole group of people, so those who despise dark skin would not tend to find any importance with matters pertaining to dark skin. The genetic inheritance of a highly melinated system is usually overlooked and not considered to be important for overall human life. The most controversial aspects of melanin research are related to human behavior. Therefore, anyone who may discuss such topics is said to be delving into controversial areas of research. To negate the positive aspects of a scientific entity (i.e., melanin) because it makes some people feel uncomfortable should never be a concern. Science is science and facts are facts. The scientific facts related to the pathology of melanin in the brain clearly indicate how significant neuromelanin or dark matter is to behavior.

In Part Two, *Dark Secrets* is presented as a biopsychosocial approach because there are societal issues such as drug addiction that are negatively affecting the African American community. Describing addiction as a disease implicates melanin because melanin has drug binding capabilities that can potentially make a person more susceptible to drug addiction. Understanding the critical scientific principles related to melanin and how behavior can be either enhanced or impaired due to melanin in the central nervous system will be addressed.

DARK MATTERS

INTRODUCTION

What does the title mean? Essentially, DARK DOES MATTER. The pigment (melanin) that provides color for living organisms and plant life is critical for the maintenance of life. It does matter if melanin is present in the human body and matters related to its presence have biological, psychological and social implications. People of African descent have been ridiculed for centuries by noncolored or less pigmented individuals because they had dark skin. Modern human and animal research, however, indicate that the pigment melanin found in dark skin and the melinated centers in the physical body are essential for proper physiological functioning. In humans, a lack of internal and external melanin can have adverse effects on the body. Therefore, dark does matter.

The topic of discussion in this volume is unique and not solely related to the dark matter in the cosmos. For the purpose of this discussion, melanin can be used interchangeably with the way dark matter is used in scientific terms. To use the expression "dark matters" is a play on words to emphasize the importance of having melanin present in the human body and to simultaneously compare melanin in the human body to the dark matter that exists in our galaxy. Based on 50 years of accumulated observations of the motions of galaxies and the expansion of the universe, most astronomers believe that as much as 90 percent of the stuff constituting the universe is dark matter (Rubin, 1998). Detecting this dark matter has helped astronomers to better comprehend the world we live in and to determine the destiny of our universe. Dark matter is important stuff, and likewise, the dark matter in our body (i.e., melanin) can determine how we function in this world as well as our fate.

If we understand that we are a microcosm of the macrocosm, then we can follow along with one of the seven Hermetic Laws of Ancient Kemet - the principle of correspondence (*As above, so below; as below, so above)*. All of these principles can be found in the ancient Kybalion, and these principles have been re-energized by the influential work of Wayne Chandler (1999) in his book, *Ancient Future*. In fact, his book on the teachings and wisdom espoused by Hermes Trismegistus has inspired me to write this second treatise on melanin. Just like the dark matter used in astronomical terms to describe the external universe, melanin is the dark matter of the internal universe (the human body).

In Part I (*Dark Matters*), alternative views on the topic and advances in melanin research will be discussed. In Chapter 1 - The Journey, we will highlight that people are physiologically different and melanin is a source of the genetic and ethnic variations. A large percentage of melanin research is on skin melanin and there is substantial evidence that skin melanin functions differently depending upon ethnicity (Chapter 2- Skin: The Large Brain). Chapter 3 - Demystifying the Melanin Molecule will provide information to better understand the hormonal influence of melanin functioning on behavior. Brain melanin or neuromelanin is much more difficult to investigate, but in Chapter 4 - The Endocrinology of Sunlight and Darkness, we will combine a discussion on the functional role between the pineal gland, melatonin and neuromelanin and how these biological entities can influence skin pigmentation and affect behavior. In Chapter 5 - Dark Matter in the Brain, we will discuss the consequences of neuromelanin pathology related to drug abuse and disease states associated with melanin and dopamine (e.g., Parkinson's Disease).

Although I am forced to use melanin/neuromelanin for descriptive purposes in this text, the reader should keep in mind that dark matter is of the essence. This dark matter has a significant role in the advancement of human functioning as well as the pathophysiology of disease. Prepare yourself for another "endarkening" experience.

T. Owens Moore
January 8, 2001

Chapter 1

The Journey

It's all around you but you can't see it...It is arguably the most important material in the universe...It will decide the fate of the universe, but we have no idea what it is. How can scientists after so many centuries, still know so little about the workings of the cosmos? As seen by the modern astronomer, that space between the planets and stars is no longer empty, and it isn't just populated by the odd dust grain or elementary particle, either. It's filled with something called dark matter..." pp.27

James Trefil (1993). Smithsonian, Vol. 24(3).

The above passage refers to dark matter in the universe, but we can similarly express the same view for the dark matter or melanin that is present in the human body; we have much to learn about both forms of dark matter. It is a oxymoron to state that we know so much about so little that eventually we will know everything about nothing. However, we are on a journey to find answers to questions that could be a mystery to our minds for another millennium. Our journey has just begun, but it is obvious that dark matter in the cosmos as well as dark matter we call melanin in the human body are the keys to open the doorway into a new cosmological perspective on what it means to be human. There is much to learn about the external universe as well as the inner universe of our human bodies.

Dark matters in the human body, and there is considerable evidence from experimental research that there are ethnic variations in melanin functioning. Unfortunately, the ethnic variations due to the presence of or lack thereof can lead to deadly consequences. For example, an obvious health risk for nonpigmented individuals is the development of a deadly form of skin cancer called melanoma.

Without melanin's protective effects, the central cause of skin cancer would be a lack of melanin to protect one from the sun's ultraviolet radiation (UV). In contrast to the apparent role of melanin in the development of skin cancer, the role of melanin may only have a contributory role in the development of hypertension in darkly pigmented individuals. There are numerous speculations as to why Blacks suffer from more hypertension compared to less pigmented individuals, but the role of melanin has received less attention.

In 1988, Pfeiffer and Mailloux hypothesized that melanin is a possible repository for heavy metals which can lead to hypertension. It is commonly believed that the occurrence of hypertension in Blacks is attributed to increased social stresses faced by Blacks. These authors suggest a more biologically relevant explanation of Black hypertension related to melanin's capabilities to absorb and attract metals and cations. In the etiology of hypertension in Blacks, cadmium, lead and copper binding to melanin have been implicated. In support of this biological model, an Italian team of investigators (Berardesca, de Rigal, Leveque and Maibach, 1991) demonstrated that ethnic differences in skin physiology exist and are mainly related to the protective role of melanin present in people with darker skin. There were marked differences between Whites, Hispanics and Blacks in stratum corneum water content and skin extensibility, recovery and elasticity.

In terms of hypertension, we understand that it is heterogenous by nature and cannot be attributed solely to any single cause. However, the link to heavy metals as well as the deficiency of other cations such as calcium, magnesium, and potassium, warrants a more nutritional approach and less reliance on current pharmacological therapy in selected cases (Pfeiffer and Maillox, 1993). These authors conclude that since melanin can be a storage bank for useful cations, it might explain the heat tolerance capacity of blacks and other dark-skinned tropical groups of people.

The advances made in the area of melanin research have led to numerous hypotheses and postulations about the extrapigmentary effects of melanin. Melanin is commonly known as the pigment on the external surface of the body which provides protection from the sun's harmful ultraviolet radiation. However, the use of modern scientific technology has generated an interest in the bioelectronic properties of melanin. Our nervous system is dependent upon electrochemical communication for normal behavioral functioning to occur, so the electrical properties of dark matter are critical for normal behavior to be expressed in organisms with complex nervous systems. Conversely, the absence of external and/or internal melanin can greatly diminish the quality of life.

Interestingly, there have been numerous articles in the popular literature that demonstrate a growing awareness for melanin's properties. In the health section of the November 2000 edition of Newsweek, it was presented that "melanin" is now available at the cosmetics counter. Dermablend's Reflection cosmetics contain a synthetic melanin, called Melasyn, that not only conceals scars and other blemishes but may help guard against skin cancer. First synthesized from the aloe vera plant by John Pawelek, a Yale skin-cancer researcher, Melasyn reflects a person's natural skin color to create an even tone. Like real melanin, Melasyn blocks UV rays and is a powerful antioxidant.

Another potent antioxidant that is also sold over the counter in health food stores is melatonin. The anti-aging effects of melatonin have also received attention from the popular media. Cowley reported in the lifestyle section of Newsweek (1995) that melatonin is a naturally cheap pill that can ease insomnia, combat jet lag, prevent pregnancy, boost the immune system, prevent cancer, extend life and prevent cells from free-radical damage. Although many of these functions are still being investigated, there is evidence that a melanin dominant biological system is more responsive to the effects of melatonin (Moore, 1996).

The pineal gland is the principal source of melatonin in the body. Much scientific data has been presented to discuss the vestigial "third eye" capabilities of the pineal gland, but you rarely find any popular media attention related to the pineal gland. In sum, the pineal is an important biological timekeeper that plays a key role in all humans, but it can have a greater influence in melanin dominant humans. In general, dark matter helps to keep our bodies youthful and to keep us connected and in rhythm with the ebb and flow of nature.

In the lifestyles section of a June 1995 issue of Jet Magazine, an article was presented to shed light on why Blacks age better than Whites. Black dermatologists are in agreement that "the elastic layer beneath the skin that keeps our skin nice and smooth does not get disrupted, broken down and degraded by the sunlight like it does in Caucasians. So our skin tends to be much smoother." In effect, there will be a lower incidence of skin cancer in Blacks compared to Whites.

It is not reverse racism to state that people of African descent are more youthful in their appearance because of dark matter, but there are some prejudiced scientists who may be offended and then neglect this area of research. In 1983, Barr stated, "General attitudes toward race may have inhibited melanin research, since melanin is the primary pigment responsible for one's skin color. Melanin (including neuromelanin) has perhaps been assumed to be only a passively acquired and thus minimally functional molecule. To downgrade the importance of melanin, however, is to overlook the significant differences between brain melanin (neuromelanin) and skin melanin properties."

Kambon (1998) bests summarizes how we should approach such criticism that melanin research from an African-centered perspective is somehow reverse racism (Jaroff, 1994). Kambon states, "...if we seek a comprehensive analysis of the melanic system, including its highly complex network of processes, which acts upon African psychological reality, the heuristic and potential value of such discourse alone would seem to outweigh, if not completely overwhelm, any intellectual discomfort over its substantive speculative aspects." It seems as though whenever non-white scholars say something provocatively about the biogenetic influences of melanin, there is criticism versus open-minded reasoning.

As expected, there have been weak (Jaroff, 1994) as well as

thorough (Willis, 1994) social critiques of melanin research in the popular literature, and the theme usually presented in these critiques is that we are all the same, so one molecule called melanin does not cause us to be different. It is true that "there are far more genetic differences among the people who make up these arbitrary constructs we call races than there are differences between races" (Willis, 1994). Ethnic variation, therefore, is a more suitable term to use versus racial classifications. It is quite apparent that conflict pertaining to the use of race is a concern primarily for western-minded, white scientists, who ironically created the confusing term. The race debate in the popular literature received attention in a special report about redefining race in America in the September 2000 issue of Newsweek. It seems as though these new race debates argued by White intellectuals coincide with the "can't we all just get along generation."

Of course we want to all get along, but to negate the biogenetic factors that dictate melanin functioning disallows a true interpretation of how genes can influence behavior. Another controversial topic is the black athlete, or should we say, "What Ever Happened to the White Athlete" (Price, 1997a, 1997b). In a special report in the Sports Illustrated magazine, a two part article was written to explore the reasons why Whites are not excelling in sports that require complex psychomotor abilities. Unsure of his place in a sports world dominated by blacks who are hungrier, harder-working and perhaps physiologically superior, the young white male is dropping out of the athletic mainstream to pursue success elsewhere (Price, 1997a). Moreover, it was questioned if the reason is in the genes. According to Price (1997b), studies have found physical differences that might help explain why blacks outperform whites in certain sports - but scientists are wary of jumping to conclusions.

Likewise, we have avoided any lengthy discussion on genetic differences that may affect athletics in this text. If there was a connection to make, it would more than likely relate to the neurotransmitter called dopamine and the interaction between dopamine and melanin in the brain. In the brain, there is a dopamine pathway that modulates pleasure (e.g., drug effects) and another pathway that modulates the motor system or movement. Any slight alteration in the interaction between dopamine and melanin can affect addiction to drugs as well as movement abilities. Dopamine is the powerful brain chemical that can get people hooked on drugs (Nash, 1997), and we have previously discussed (Moore, 1995) the possibility that there may be a genetic sensitivity issue to explain why drugs affect people differently. Similarly, if dopamine affects drug addiction and dopamine is also important for movement, then we can speculate that the composition of the nervous system is a major source of ethnic differences in athletic ability. As stated earlier, it is suggested that brain melanin is genetically programmed to function at different capacities depending upon a person's overall genetic capacity to produce melanin.

Dopamine is one of many neurochemicals found in the brain, but we must consider its importance because of its overlapping role in drug addiction, Parkinson's disease and schizophrenia. Dopamine is widely distributed throughout the brain, and it accounts for about half of the total catecholamines in the brain (Sian, et al., 1999). The two major dopamine pathways are the nigrostriatal (movement) and mesolimbic (emotion) pathways. Interestingly, over 80% of dopamine in the brain is found in the basal ganglia, where the initiation of movement is generated. Along with hard work and practice, dopamine-melanin interactions in the basal ganglia may be the biological source for the excellence achieved by Black athletes in sporting events requiring complex psychomotor skills.

In addition to dopamine as a separate biological entity, we cannot underestimate the importance of a dopamine-melanin interaction for normal behavioral functioning. We have provided evidence that dark matter or neuromelanin coexists within dopamine producing cells to provide protection against toxic agents, to enhance movement-oriented tasks, and to positively affect ones emotional experience. Therefore, dark matter in the brain is critical for the normal expression of mental perceptions, memory capabilities, and psychomotor skills. From the experimental research reviewed in this text, it appears as though dark matter is present in the brain to enhance the speed of nerve impulses, to transform physical energy from one physical state into a signal the nervous system can detect, and to provide protection to delicate brain cells from neurotoxic substances.

Our discussion has been on both the external pigmentary effects of melanin in the skin as well as the internal presence of melanin in the body, specifically the nervous system. In both locations, melanin dominant individuals have a biological system full of antioxidant technology to keep the body looking and feeling younger as well as protecting the nervous system from neurotoxicity. If overburdened, however, melanin functioning may be detrimental and contribute to the formation of neurodegenerative disorders. Our diet is one very important factor where we can assist in the maintenance of positive mental and physical health as well as prevent the inadvertent destruction of cells which cause disease. The consumption of vitamins E, D and C are only a few dietary factors mentioned that can help to keep our bodies functioning efficiently as we age.

To conclude, DARK DOES MATTER in the process of improving the quality of life. How much time we spend in the sun, and what we consume and digest over the years can have an accumulative effect on the body. Smelling, sniffing and swallowing substances are common ways that toxic agents can gain entry to our biological systems. Obviously, we cannot monitor everything we are exposed to because too frequently, the exposure is inadvertent in the form of pesticides, ingredients in food, the consumption of recreational drugs, and from daily doses of the sun. Toxicity develops over time and the body attempts to fight back with its natural antioxidants (melanin and melatonin). It is recommended that we eat as much sun-enriched foods as possible and also allow the sun to be our friend and not our enemy. So eat right, stay fit and let almighty RA bathe us with the life force it generates.

Chapter 2

Skin: The Large Brain

A provocative perspective on skin functioning relates to the skin as a "large brain." As a living and breathing element, the skin is of the utmost importance to human life. It encases all of the vital functions of the body and it is in direct contact with the external world. The brain inside the cranium guides the internal mechanisms of the body. Similarly, the skin can be considered the brain that controls the external mechanisms of the body.

The skin mainly serves as a protective surface against the earth's elements. For example, water is repelled by the unique structure of the skin's surface and air is interchanged to keep our body temperature ambient. From a biological perspective, the skin does not only function as a covering for the body; the skin actually functions as a large organ that can physiologically respond to external stimuli. Moreover, it appears as though the skin can respond to neurochemicals released from the brain and also generate these chemicals locally in the skin. In other words, there are biochemical mechanisms that exist in the skin that appear very similar to many processes that occur in the brain. It is not so important that we think of the skin as a brain, but that we understand the similarities between the brain and the skin.

BRAIN AND SKIN SIMILARITIES

Tyrosine, an essential amino acid, is the first similarity that can be made to connect the brain and the skin. In the brain, for example, tyrosine is an important precursor molecule for the biosynthesis of neurotransmitters. In the skin, tyrosine is an important component in the formation of melanin. The enzymatic conversion of tyrosine is the critical factor which will determine the formation of neurotransmitters in the brain or melanin in the skin. *Tyrosine hydroxylase* is the enzyme needed in the brain and *tyrosinase* is the enzyme needed in the skin. Without the presence of tyrosinase, there would be no external pigment to provide protection against the ultraviolet radiation of the sun. Albinism would be the genetic abnormality observed if no tyrosinase was present in a person's genetic structure. In addition, the absence of melanin in the skin could contribute to the aging process that occurs from exposure to environmental pollutants.

Tyrosine is needed to synthesize common biological substrates (i.e., catecholamines and melanin) in both the brain and the skin. As a final common pathway, some researchers (Iyengar and Misra, 1988) have speculated that tyrosine's conversion into catecholamines (dopamine, norepinephrine and epinephrine) and then melanin could occur in both the skin and the brain. Tyrosine leads to the biosynthesis of melanin in the skin, but it is not commonly believed that tyrosine is specific for synthesizing neurotransmitters in the skin. In the brain, there is some speculation that melanin is a "waste product" from catecholamine synthesis, perhaps forming neuromelanin. Since we know that melanin has many important functions (see Moore, 1995), we could not conclude that it is a "waste product."

Since dark does matter, we can view melanin as more than just a skin pigment. Think of the skin as a "large brain" that can secrete hormones from specialized cells in a similar way that the brain secretes hormones. Melanin in the skin is a hormone released from specialized cells called melanocytes. Hormones are defined as chemical messengers that are released from cells in one area of the body to stimulate cells in another area of the body. The stimulation of melanocytes from stimuli such as light, however, causes a local effect. The local effect is an increase in skin pigmentation where the melanocytes are located. The biosynthesis of melanin is further needed to regulate other physiological processes such as vitamin D synthesis. If melanin is unable to perform its physiological role as a hormonal control of vitamin D synthesis and calcium absorption, physical abnormalities will exist. For example, older females who lack melanin can develop osteoporosis and a lack of vitamin D in young people can cause rickets to develop (Holick, 1985).

INTRINSIC PIGMENTARY FACTORS

Historically, ultraviolet radiation from the sun has been the sole factor associated with darkening human skin. It makes sense because the sun bathes the skin and the skin is then responsive to the sun's powerfully effects. Therefore, tanning from the sun has been the main focus on how the skin can darken. The skin, however, is also responsive to hormonal influences that are independent of the sun's effects. Research from animal studies has demonstrated that pigmentation is regulated by several hormonal influences (see Bagnara and Hadley, 1973) and not only UV radiation.

In humans, pigment cell researchers have been hesitant to attribute a functional role for melanin beyond a sunscreen. It is worth noting that most pigment cell researchers who have investigated the functional role of melanin have historically been nonpigmented in their external appearance. You can understand the difficulty of trying to interpret the complex nature of skin pigmentation when the phenomenon is far removed from the interpreter's reality. Therefore, we have had a lack of interest and a slow progression towards establishing a hormonal connection with melanin functioning. Current experimental evidence exposes the complexity and sheds light on the fact that the skin is a "large brain."

It is not suggested that the skin has the same thinking capabilities as the brain in our skulls. The brain in our skull is the most complex entity in the universe. Making the statement that the skin is a "large brain" relates to similar chemicals (e.g., POMC, ACTH and MSH) that are detected in the two organs. Although a detailed description of these chemicals has been provided (Moore, 1995 see Chapter 5), we will further discuss their importance in the next chapter. The point to highlight is that these neurochemicals have multiple functions and the production of POMC, ACTH and MSH in the skin may suggest a far greater role beyond the stimulation of melanocytes.

In 1995, I only emphasized MSH and 8-methoxy psoralen as potential chemicals that can darken the skin without the effects of sunlight. There are, however, many more chemicals that can be found in any Physician's Desk Reference. It has been known that pigmentation is to a certain extent under hormonal control (Le Douarin and Kalcheim, 1999), and animal studies have shown that there are numerous hormones that can act as potent regulators of pigmentation. In amphibians, manifestation of adult pigmentation is regulated by thyroid hormones (Bagnara and Hadley, 1973). In addition, prolactin has long been known to play a major role in bringing about the various changes occurring in second metamorphosis in newts (Grant, 1961). Sex hormones are responsible for the onset of adult bright pigmentation in amphibians and other vertebrates as well (Le Douarin and Kalcheim, 1999). The most common pigmentary factor, however, is melanocyte-stimulating hormone (MSH). Multiple roles for MSH beyond melanogenesis have been reviewed elsewhere (Moore, 1995).

MELANOCORTIN RECEPTORS

If the skin is responsive to chemicals, then there must be sites in the skin where reactions occur. It has been found in the recent years that MSH activity on pigmentation is mediated in humans by the melanocortin-1 receptor (MC1R), a seven transmembrane G protein-coupled receptor expressed by melanocytes. Activation of MC1R produces elevated levels of intracellular cAMP (Mountjoy et al., 1992) and triggers the pathway leading to melanin synthesis.

Classically, POMC-derived peptides are considered as pituitary hormones. However, they have been shown to be produced also in the mammalian brain and in a variety of peripheral tissues, including the gastrointestinal tract, the reproductive organs, and in cells of the immune system (see Wintzen and Gilchrest, 1996, for a review). More recently, POMC-derived peptides have been found in mammalian epidermal cells, including human keratinocytes (Slominski et al., 1992; Farooqui et al., 1993) and even in melanocytes. POMC transcripts were detected first in human and rodent melanoma cell lines and more recently also in UV-stimulated human melanocytes. All these cells were found to contain alpha-MSH and ACTH immunoreactivity (reviewed by Wintzen and Gilchrest, 1996).

In an attempt to address the findings that cultured melanocytes are unresponsive to peptides, researchers in a 1994 study in the United Kingdom demonstrated that cultured melanocytes respond to MSH peptides and ACTH (Hunt et al., 1994). The cultured tissue was processed from human melanocytes isolated from foreskins and breast-reduction skin from Caucasian and Asian subjects. In sum, ACTH affected morphology and stimulated melanogenesis and tyrosinase activity in human melanocytes. The cells were sensitive to the concentration, however. The dose-response curves for ACTH were biphasic, and the melanocytes responded to lower concentrations of ACTH than MSH peptides, similar to those normally present in human plasma. The receptor content of the cultures would also be a critical factor determining the responsiveness of cultured melanocytes to peptide exposure. Furthermore, one can take note that darkly melinated skin (i.e., Black) would probably be more responsive than the skin of the Caucasian and Asian subjects used in the Hunt et al. study.

Although melanin in the skin appears to be a simple layer of pigment, the epidermal melanin unit is rather complex (Fitzpatrick and Breathnach, 1963). Melanosomes synthesized within melanocytes are delivered to surrounding keratinocytes and spread to epidermal melanocytes. More complexity is found where the receptor sites are located on both epidermal and keratinocytes. Jiang et al. (1996) revealed that almost every melanocyte possesses melanocortin receptors as visualized by scanning electron microscopy. In fact, both epidermal and keratinocytes have been cultured *in vitro* and are said to possess MSH or melanocortin receptors (MCRs). Since MSH can function as a neurotransmitter in the brain, certain neurons would be expected to also possess MSH receptors (Hruby et al., 1996).

The receptors for alpha-MSH and ACTH have been cloned (Chhajlani and Wikberg, 1992; Mountjoy et al., 1992). There are five different subtypes of the MCR (Hadley et al., 1996) and probably more to be discovered for ACTH. As suggested by Hruby et al. (1996), some of the MCR subtypes are in the brain. For example, MC3R expression has been detected in the brain and periphery and MC4R is expressed in a wide distribution of peripheral tissues. Although some researchers (Pawelek et al., 1992) have suggested that humans apparently lack a pituitary source of melanotropic peptide, there is accumulating evidence that the skin itself is a source of a melanocortin that may regulate integumental melanogenesis, particularly in response to ultraviolet radiation. Furthermore, the research detailing the complexity of MCRs highlights our discussion on drug addiction in Part Two of this text (*Dark Secrets*). In other words, drugs can interact with the skin and potentially affect the physiological response to the drug. Altering the receptor physiology in the skin could make a drug effect last longer or cause an adverse reaction. Drug addiction might result from an altered receptor physiology, and in this case, the receptors would be MCRs.

THE CELLULAR KA

As previously stated, the epidermal melanin unit is complex (Fig. 1). An innovative approach we can use to provide some clarity and to describe the structure of the melanocyte requires a minor digression into ancient African terminology. For example, the cellular KA is a physical analogy used to describe the structure and function of the melanocyte in the skin. First, KA is an ancient Kemetic term that describes the physical part of the soul. KA is represented as two vertically extended arms in Metu Neter or hieroglyphic symbology. If you visualize the actual structure of a melanocyte, it has a body containing the nucleus and two arms extending to the surface of the skin. Melanosomes migrate up the arms to provide the even pigmentation we see on our skin. The arms are extended outward as if they are reaching for the sun's rays. If we speak in Kemetic terms, the cellular KA is reaching out to be bathed by almighty RA (i.e., sun).

As we return to modern scientific terms, the structure of melanocytes could be considered as nerve cells located in the skin. The extending arms of the cellular KA are actually dendrites or the receiving portion of the nerve cell. Some researchers have suggested that melanocytes are actually neuroendocrine cells that produce dopamine and noradrenaline besides melanin (Iyengar and Misra, 1988). It is provocative to suggest that the skin can produce neurotransmitters because it highlights a perceptive role of the skin. When people say they feel something or experience a sixth sense, perhaps the "large brain" is responding to the environment. It is difficult to say our skin is conscious, but it has some of the brain chemicals that do affect our mental awareness.

Exposure to the sun may be underestimated by many but the energy from the sun should be a daily quest. Since UV dependent pigmentation is associated with POMC production in skin (Iyengar, 1995), sunlight apparently does much more than increase the melanin content in the skin. The pleasurable feelings associated with exposure to the sun may be due to a higher circulation of neurotransmitters in the body. Knowing that the skin has the ability to generate chemicals that are normally associated with the brain suggests a very important role for touch. The sensitivity of a touch and a hug may stimulate a hormonal release of neurotransmitters directly from the skin. The neuroendocrine response of a melanocyte from stimuli such as a touch or a hug might stimulate a euphoric response.

Another provocative finding from a team of Japanese researchers (Maeda, Naganuma, Fukuda, Matsunaga and Tomita, 1996) demonstrated that steroid hormones can also stimulate melanogenesis in cultured cells from Japanese males. Normal human melanocytes in culture became enlarged and dendritic after a 2-day incubation with either the pituitary (beta-MSH, alpha-MSH, ACTH, FSH and LH) or the ovarian (estradiol, estriol and progesterone) hormones. Under the same experimental conditions, pituitary hormones also increased both the tyrosinase activity and tyrosinase-related protein-1 (TRP-1) while ovarian hormones increased TRP-1 but not tyrosinase activity. These data demonstrated that pituitary and ovarian hormones possibly induced hyperpigmentation of the skin by stimulating the melanogenesis in epidermal melanocytes. The increased pigmentation found in various regions of a pregnant woman's body is possibly due to both MSH and ovarian hormones (Fig. 2).

According to the findings presented in this chapter, dark does matter and melanin is more than a colorful pigment. Hue is certainly important for individual variation, but melanin does more than just make us colorful people. For instance, the liver, pancreas, gall bladder and kidney are organs that have multiple functions, and so we can view the skin as more than a body protectant. The skin can perform a host of functions that can keep the individual looking youthful. For instance, sometimes it is easy to tell the health status of an individual by observing the appearance of their skin. During childhood, people often talk about having skin as smooth as a baby. During puberty, increased circulation of hormones may cause acne. As one ages and consumes too many sweets or toxic substances (e.g., alcohol and drugs), the skin may form bumps and rashes. Also, the formation of eczema may result from a poor diet. Melanin may function as protection against these negative consequences and help to prolong the beauty of ones' external appearance.

In sum, we can conclude that melanin is more than just a pigment and the skin is more than just an outer covering. In the next chapter, we will become more "endarkened" by learning new perspectives on melanin functioning.

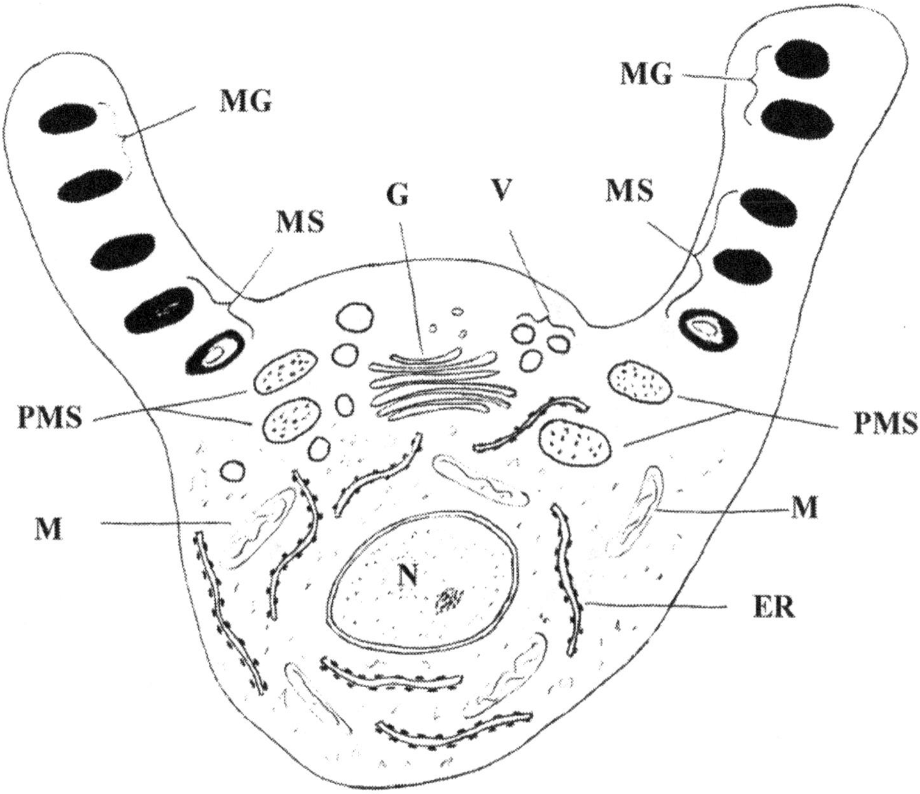

Figure 1 - Diagram of a melanocyte, showing melanin granules in various stages of development. The polypeptides that eventually become 'tyrosinase' are synthesized in small granules, transferred, perhaps along the endoplasmic reticulum (ER), to Golgi area (G), and condensed into 'protyrosinase'. In the Golgi area, protyrosinase is separated into small units, each of which becomes surrounded by a membranous envelope (V). Within each envelope, the protyrosinase molecules become oriented forming a ' premelanosome' (PMS). The protyrosinase then becomes active, i.e., becomes tyrosinase, melanin biosynthesis begins and the particle is known as a 'melanosome' (MS). As melanin accumulates, the melanosome is eventually transformed into a dense particle, the 'melanin granule' (MG) in which no tyrosinase activity can be detected.

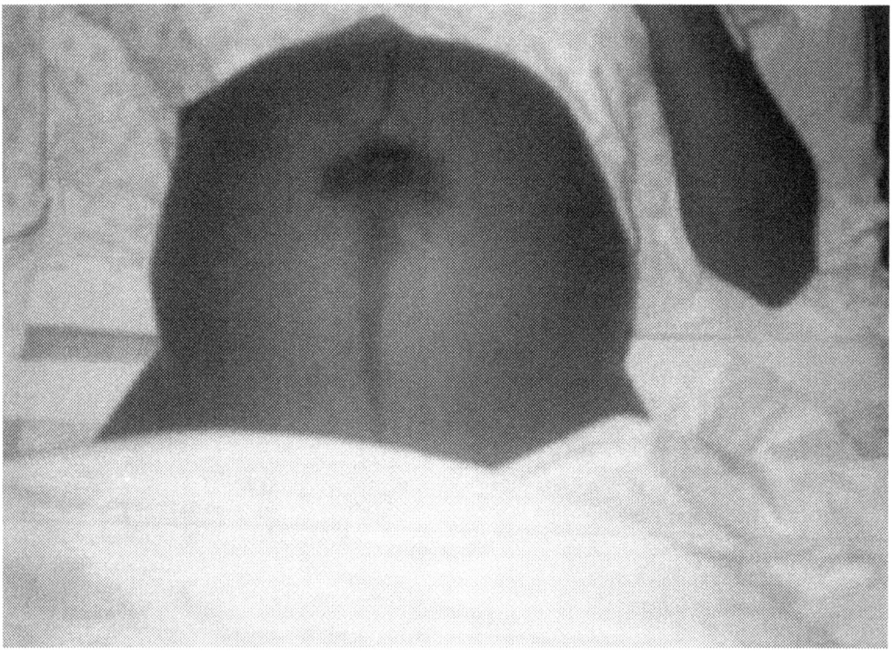

Figure 2 - The stomach of a woman just prior to birth. Pigmentation is regulated by hormonal influences. Melanocyte-stimulating hormone (MSH) secreted from the pituitary gland stimulates a distinct area of melanocytes on the surface of the stomach to produce high levels of melanin around the belly button.

Chapter 3

Demystifying the Melanin Molecule

With all of the advancement in space exploration, we are discovering new phenomena about our universe everyday. For example, new planets in our galaxy have been found, other galaxies have been detected and dark matter continues to be the cosmic mesh that is holding the external world together. Astrophysicists have made significant advances in space exploration with the use of shuttle missions into space and high tech telescopes. Similarly, biomedical scientist are now looking deeper into the brain and body with advanced technology to discover new perspectives on the inner workings of our human body or internal universe. The human body also possesses its own dark matter (melanin) and there has been considerable advancements pertaining to melanin's effects on the human body.

NEUROMELANIN AND THE MIND

F.E. Barr (1983) published the first synthesis of extensive research into melanin and an integrative process theory of living systems. The purpose of this extensive review was to focus scientific attention on a relatively neglected but strategically significant area of research (specifically neuromelanin). Over 700 hundred articles related to the science of melanin were synthesized into a major hypothesis that melanin functions as the most significant organizational molecule in living systems through its effective *in vivo* control of the vital and diverse covalent modifications crucial for both physiological and psychological activity.

Using DNA and RNA as a theoretical base, Barr discussed how these nucleic acids exert an activational programming control over the numerous passively activated, functionally dynamic proteins. After being actively programmed, these proteins (e.g., enzymes) may actually be able to evoke their dynamic programmed responses *in vitro*. The same "activational-static" classification given to DNA may be applied to melanin for *in vitro* studies.

Barr hypothesized that melanin has evolved in its "activational-static" organizational capacity from the regulation of molecular-cellular-tissue systems in lower organisms to an advanced CNS neuromelanin-neuroendocrine network in higher organisms and a subsequent self-conscious mental capacity in humans. In addition, melanin's potential ability to integrate and organize the neuroendocrine system, and its ability to do so by affecting electrochemical communication in the nervous system would seem to necessitate the consideration of neuromelanin as a serious candidate for linking "mind and brain" (Barr, 1983).

In an attempt to depoliticize neuromelanin research, Barr states, "One's neuromelanin does not correlate clearly with one's skin melanin, in either known formative mechanisms, gross amounts, or major functions. While the internal molecular arrangements and diffuse interconnections of one's neuromelanin-monoamine network may vary uniquely with each individual, such variations in one's neuromelanin do not correlate (in any obvious way) with one's skin color (whether white, red, yellow, black, brown, or albino)."

Barr (1983) clearly set the bar or standard for academic scholarship so high that no other source of literature has come close to meet the standards of this lengthy but condensed review of melanin. Dynamic and provocative ideas should never be shunned because of politics. Scientific explorations should be for the advancement of life, so scientists should embrace Barr's ideas with fervor.

JEWEL POOKRUM HYPOTHESIS

One of the most dynamic African American scholars to present a discourse on melanin and its significant role in the human body is Jewel Pookrum (1993). She is an internationally recognized scientists who has lectured throughout the country on a multitude of topics related to health and nutrition. With her research experience and medical background, she has provided us with fascinating ideas in her thought provoking lectures.

In a synopsis, she provides scientific evidence that the quality of life is greatly enhanced with the presence of melanin. In her book, *Vitamins and Minerals From A to Z* (1993), she begins her discussion on the importance of considering ethnicity in the context of health promotion. A discussion on ethnicity lays the groundwork for how to enhance life for melanin-dominant people. Next, she provides the reader with a very concise but thorough chapter on what melanin is and how it functions in the human body. Moreover, she provides a chapter on the relationship between light and good health. She does an excellent job introducing the reader to the pineal gland, a light transducing organ that is linked to melanin functioning. She concludes with a lengthy description of vitamins and minerals and how they can be used to promote health in melanin-dominant individuals.

As a scholar, Pookrum's well rounded background can single handedly demystify all concepts related to the melanin molecule. Her scientific interpretations of melanin properties are based on facts that have been supported by experimental research. She provides numerous examples of melanin properties that reveal the electrical nature of melanin. For example, melanin exhibits varying types of electrical charges and binding properties responsible for its great electromagnetic and electric activity. Melanin responds to and absorbs light, sound and electrical energy. In addition, melanin can bind and release most of the known elements of earth. These elements include certain minerals such as calcium, iron, zinc, potassium, and sodium, which are essential for numerous bodily functions.

The connection we made in Chapter 2 in which we called the skin a "large brain" or an extrasensory perceptive organ is pertinent to the views espoused by Pookrum (1993). In her discussion on the nervous system, she mentions that melanin is necessary for proper receptivity of energy imparted to our bodies from the external environment. In terms of external stimuli, light is not just the color sensation perceived by the eye, light is also heat, radiation, laser waves, cosmic waves, radio waves, TV waves, magnetism, and electrical currents. Due to melanin's tremendous capacity to absorb these forms of light and use them as energy sources to recharge itself and the cells in which it is located, melanin's strategic relationship with the central nervous system also gives us the capacity to immediately know what is happening to us within our external environment. This gives human beings great ability to be aware of their internal environment, and constantly be recharged and regenerated from interacting with the external environment.

In sum, Pookrum has helped to endarken our understanding of melanin's diverse effects on the human body. Her views should be studied intensely if one is to mentally grasp the cosmic connection of this dark matter as well as the cellular mechanisms that help the nervous system to function at an optimal level. The nervous system is a very important part of our discussion, so the next section will explore the origin of melanin in the nervous system and follow with the ionic mechanism that can be mediated by melanin.

THE CREATION OF DARK MATTER

Melanins are unique, irregular, amorphous pigmented polymers widely distributed throughout the human body. During embryonic development in the womb of darkness, melanins originate from a distinct layer of cells called the ectoderm. The ectoderm explodes like a "Big Bang" and further divides into the prospective neural tube, the prospective neural crest and the prospective epidermal layer. Melanin is distributed to various parts of the internal universe by these specialized cell groups, and it is amazing how the tiny mass of cells in the ectoderm can transform into a miniature solar system.

After conceptualizing the principles of the Kybalion (see Chandler, 1999), a very clear analogy can be made in reference to the structure of our galaxy (The Milky Way) and the formation of the human body. Powerful instruments such as the Hubble and the Keck telescope have revealed that our galaxy has spiraling arms that swirl placidly. However, infrared detectors have revealed that the galactic center or core is a violent storm of exploding stars and roiling gas, all circling a hungry black hole. Stars moving in the galactic core orbit as fast as .5 percent the speed of light, or about 900 miles per second. Scientists speculated that whatever entity was keeping stars in that fast of an orbit had to have a mass of about 2.5 million suns. The tight orbit of the nearest stars meant that all that mass was packed into a relatively tiny space. Only one entity fits those specs and the law of physics: a black hole (Freedman, 1998). Likewise, melanin is the black hole at the center of the embryo that can harness energy and give rise to a new life. For the birth of a human being, imagine what could be revealed if there was a miniature Hubble in the bubble of the belly?

Without the miniature telescope, developmental biologists have still managed to determine the body parts that are formed from ectodermal cells. The *neural tube* is differentiated into a) brain, b) the spinal cord, c) posterior pituitary gland, d) the optic vesicles, and e) the motor nerves that originate in the ventral portion of the neural tube and innervate muscles. The *neural crest* derivatives consist of cells that migrate to distant parts of the body. These migrating cells form sensory nerves and ganglia, which receive impulses from the following sites: 1) sense organs; 2) autonomic ganglia; 3) the adrenal medulla; 4) all of the pigmented retina cells, which are derived from the neural tube; 5) the cartilages in the voice box and head; and 6) some of the ectodermal muscles. The *epidermal layer* can be divided into cells derived from epidermal thickening and those derived from the rest of the epidermis. The thick epidermal derivatives include some of the cranial nerves, the lens of the eye, the olfactory structures, the inner ear, and taste buds. The remainder of the epidermis forms the following structures: the anterior pituitary gland; the hair and nails; the linings of the mouth and anus; and the outer layer of the skin.

Melanocytes in the skin are like specialized nerve cells which contain melanin. Since cells containing melanin have properties similar to nerve cells, we can begin to understand the extrasensory perceptive abilities of the skin and the bioelectrical effects that are reported in melinated tissue . When it is stated that melanin can bind and release ions such as calcium, sodium and potassium (Pookrum, 1993), it implies that melinated cells can mediate some very important physiological mechanisms.

IONIC INTERCHANGE

The control of cells by intricate cellular mechanisms is the first stimulation needed before a cell can exert its biological effects. Small gates or channels reside on cells to assist in the stimulation of a cell, for example, prior to the release of a hormone. Without ions such as potassium, calcium, sodium and chloride, it would be difficult for our nervous system to function. Pharmacological treatment with drugs that can stimulate as well as inhibit ion flow provide experimental evidence for the importance of having ions to conduct normal biological functions. Melanin's bioelectrical properties can help to absorb these charged particles and subsequently increase cellular activity.

There is evidence suggesting that calcium can be involved in the control of melanogenesis (Fuller, 1987), possibly by a calmodulin-dependent mechanism (Buffey et al., 1991; Hill et al., 1989), but the pathways for calcium entry into the melanocyte are not well understood. Nilius et al. (1990) described the properties of voltage-activated potassium channels in a human melanoma cell line. These authors suggested that such channels are involved in the control of cell proliferation (Nilius and Wohlrab, 1992).

In the first electrophysiological recordings of human melanocytes using the patch-clamp technique, Ekmehag et al.(1994) demonstrated that human melanocytes, in addition to two types of potassium channels similar to potassium channels in melanoma cells, are equipped with voltage-dependent and TTX-sensitive sodium channels (TTX is a toxin that can shut down sodium functioning). If the sodium current does not flow, then there is no activity in the nervous system.

Ekmehag et al. used human melanocytes from extracted foreskins obtained after circumcision. The study was performed in

Sweden, so it is likely the subjects were all Caucasian. According to scientist such as Pookrum (1993), the ethnicity of the subjects is very important because the results could be dependent on the level of pigmentation in the subject's skin. Darker skin may absorb more ions and perhaps contain higher levels of sodium channels. The sodium current described by Ekmehag et al. shares many of the characteristics of voltage-dependent sodium currents in muscle, secretory cells and nerve cells (Hille, 1992). According to Ekmehag et al., one could consider the possibility that the sodium channels in melanocytes simply are "remnants" reflecting the origin of the cells in the neural crest.

INNER EAR MELANIN

Similar to the melanocytes in the skin, inner ear melanin is also derived from the neural crest. The greater one's genetic capacity to produce melanin in the skin would imply a higher content of melanin in other locations, for example, the inner ear. Essentially, the relationship between pigmentation and hearing has been known for more than a century. I have already reviewed inner ear melanin and its role in human behavior (Moore, 1995), but an intriguing article written by Masayoshi Tachibana (1999) has provided more clarity on the relationship between sound and melanocytes.

In this review, data from genetically mutated animals (albino rats, albino guinea pigs and black-eyed white mutant mice) and a rare human genetic disease (VKH) were used to describe a functional role for melanocytes in the inner ear. Vogt-Koyanagi-Harada (VKH) is an uncommon systemic disorder characterized by panuveitis associated with disorders of skin, inner ear and leptomeninges; it occurs almost exclusively in darkly pigmented individuals (Rao et al., 1995). It is tempting to conceive that this disease is an autoimmune disease whose targets are melanocyte-specific proteins (Tachibana, 1999).

Cytotoxic T lymphocytes were shown to kill melanocytes recognizing MART-1 melanoma antigen in patients with VKH disease (Sugita et al., 1996), and melanin-laden macrophages were found in cerebrospinal fluid of patients with VKH disease (Nakamura et al.,

1996). Regardless of the pathogenesis, the common histopathological finding in the affected skin and eye of VKH diseases is T-cell-mediated inflammation around melanocytes (Kahn et al., 1993; Okada et al., 1996). Since a high incidence of hearing impairment, supposedly acquired, is reported in VKH disease (Kimura et al., 1996), it is conceivable that melanocytes in the cochlea may also be targeted by cytotoxic T cells and damaged in patients with VKH disease. According to Tachibana (1999), sound needs melanocytes to hear and these data indicate that healthy melanocytes are required for normal hearing.

When human or animals were exposed to intense sound, the hearing function often deteriorated, temporarily or permanently. Some studies related decreased iris or skin pigmentation to severity of noise-induced temporary threshold shift (Barrenas and Lingren, 1990) or permanent hearing loss (Tota and Bocci, 1967; Hood et al., 1976; Carter, 1980; Carter et al., 1981) in humans. Conlee et al. (1986, 1988) measured cochlear microphonics before and after exposure in albino and pigmented guinea pigs and concluded that albino guinea pigs are more susceptible to the ototoxic effects of high intensity noise than pigmented guinea pigs. Lower susceptibility to noise in pigmented cochlea may be explained by melanin's ability to scavenge reactive oxygen species (Bustamante et al., 1993), which appear after exposure to noise (Yamane et al., 1995). *In vivo* administration of free radical scavenger has been shown to attenuate noise-induced hair cell damage (Yamasoba et al., 1999).

We are all familiar with the "bass heads" who blast their music in the confined space of their car. It is not only irritating to others nearby, but it is causing permanent damage to the bass head. Blasting loud music may seem harmless to the bass head, but knowing the delicate nature of the hair cell structure reveals that the bass head will be joining the future hearing aid society. Inner ear melanin may lessen the damage, but the impending toxicity formed over time will be detrimental.

Toxicity in the ear can also be caused by drugs. Melanin binds many chemicals, including ototoxic drugs such as aminoglycoside antibiotics, and is considered to be a protective chemical filter. Melanin may protect tissue from potentially harmful substances by binding and slowly releasing the agents in low, nontoxic concentrations (Larsson, 1993). Consistent with this hypothesis, Conlee and colleagues (1994, 1995) found that pigmented guinea pigs are less susceptible to gentamicin ototoxicity than albino guinea pigs.

OTHER FACTORS INVOLVED IN THE MELANIZATION PROCESS

Light primarily from the sun is the major progenitor of external melanization. Whether external or internal, the occurrence of melanin is to protect tissue from the damaging effects of toxic substances. However, there appears to be melanin production that does not depend on ultraviolet radiation. The male penis is an external body site that is darker than other parts of the human anatomy, but it does not receive direct sunlight. The dark pigment that appears on the surface of a cut piece of fruit or the dark pigment that occurs on a healing flesh wound are other melanization effects that do not depend on the sun. Moreover, the extensive melanization occurring in specific cells in the course of certain pathological conditions, such as melanoma or Parkinson's Disease, are reasons to suggest that melanization can occur independent of sun exposure.

As part of the melanization process, enzymes play a very key role in the conversion of biological substrates in the melanin pathway. For example, tyrosinase has been the key enzyme involved in the conversion of tyrosine into skin melanin. No tyrosinase was detected in the brain (Carstam et al., 1991), so melanization in the brain is probably due to tyrosine hydroxylase. Current research has revealed that eumelanogenesis of human skin melanocytes requires at least three enzymes: tyrosinase, tyrosine-related-protein 1 (TRP-1), and tyrosine-related-protein 2 (TRP-2) (Tobin et al., 1994; Kippenberger et al., 1996). The discovery of these additional enzymes has added to the complexity of melanization. The presence of TRP-1 and TRP-2 may help to determine the production of different pigments.

According to Kippenberger et al. (1996), they seem to be involved in the modulation of the quality and quantity of melanins. Kippenberger et al. studied melanocytes isolated from human fetal back skin and keratinocytes from human abdominal skin. They used RT-PCR to investigate the transcription of all three enzymes in both keratinocytes and melanocytes. In agreement with other research (Tobin et al., 1994), transcription of all three enzymes was positively detected. It is suspected that mutations of the TRP-1 gene in humans can lead to a tyrosinase positive albinism (Boissy et al., 1996), so these data have significant implications.

Tobin and colleagues (1994) studied these three enzymes in four different skin types. For each protein, the numbers of positively stained melanocytes were similar in all subjects studied irrespective of skin type. Following five daily suberythemal doses of UVB, the melanocytes were larger, more dendritic, and increased in number. With TRP-1 and TRP-2, the increase in number in response to UVB was unrelated to skin type or melanin content. With tyrosinase, however, there was a much greater increase in skin types III and IV(dark skin) than in skin types I and II (light skin). Skin types with higher melanin content had enhanced numbers of tyrosinase-positive melanocytes and increased staining intensity. This increase in tyrosinase could be related to the greater levels of eumelanin found in skin types III and IV, and this is in keeping with the view that higher levels of tyrosinase are associated with the production of eumelanin than pheomelanin.

Besides the discovery of tyrosine-related-proteins, there is a new chapter to be written as we attempt to understand melanin functioning. Another discovery relates to the formation of melanins from opioid peptides (Rosei, 1996). *In vitro* biochemical studies using mushroom and sepia tyrosinase were able to give rise to synthetic melanins. For several years, Rosei and colleagues have been engaged in the investigation of novel model pathways dealing with *in vitro* melanin production. In regard to additional enzymes, they have demonstrated that, in the presence of hydrogen peroxide, lipoxygenase and xanthine oxidase can produce eumelanins or pheomelanins *in vitro* (Rosei et al., 1994, 1995). There is circumstantial evidence that some of the enzymes mentioned above are active in melanin synthesis *in vivo* during aging or in the course of Parkinson's Disease (Adams and Odunze, 1991).

Opioid peptides were chosen because they represent a large class among animal peptides that can be divided into three groups: enkephalins, endorphins and dynorphins. Each of these small peptides is derived from a larger peptide called pro-opiomelanocortin (POMC). The opioid peptides are known as a group of neurotransmitters and neurohormones sharing the common feature of an amino terminal tyrosine residue that is essential for binding to the receptors (Rada et al., 1986). According to Rosei (1996), any peptide both natural and synthetic that presents an amino terminal tyrosine residue is able to generate a peptide-melanin upon tyrosinase action. The sequence of reactions that is postulated to explain the oxidation of enkephalins and related peptides by tyrosinase essentially repeats the Mason-Raper Pathway.

Though it has long been known that natural melanins occur as complex structures, melanin pigments were thought to be only formed by the oxidation of simple molecules such as amines, aminoacids or dihydroxyindoles (Ito, 1993; Prota, 1992). The possible existence *in vivo* of opiomelanins, and any physiological functions they may have is another possible way melanins are produced.

We do know, however, that opioid peptides can exert opiate-like effects and their role as neurotransmitters and hormones has been demonstrated (e.g., Beaumon and Hughes, 1979; Huda et al., 1984). Both enkephalins and enkephalin receptors are ubiquitous and have, in particular, been found in the brain (Cooper et al., 1991) and in melanoma cell culture (Slominski et al., 1991; Zagon et al. 1996), where tyrosinase expression is well documented (Prota, 1992). The proximity of opioidergic and dopaminergic fibers in substantia nigra and locus coeruleus neurons has been ascertained (Zamir et al., 1984); and the great number of opioid receptors in these locations (Cooper et al., 1991) encourages the suspicion that opiomelanins are involved in the process of Parkinsonian melanization.

In sum, the discovery of opiomelanins is another scientific advancement that allows us to look deeper into the role of melanin in the body. We have addressed several ideas in this chapter that are centered on empirical research, so the melanin molecule should not be considered a mystery substance. It is a very essential molecule that can provide structure to our lives from birth to death.

The next chapter will continue to focus on the nervous system. The role of the pineal gland, melatonin and melanin (specifically neuromelanin) will be presented. The pineal gland is a light transducing neuroanatomical structure, and it produces a hormone called melatonin. Neuromelanin is distinctly different from melatonin but it is also found in the brain. They are popular topics related to melanin that deserve considerable attention.

Chapter 4

The Endocrinology of Sunlight and Darkness

The energy generated from the sun has been a major factor affecting the evolution of human beings. The sun is like a nuclear power plant that emits power for our entire solar system. We are connected to the sun during every minute of our existence, and the continued presence of the sun's radiance has life-promoting properties as well as death-inducing effects. Human beings have evolved to be the masters of this universe because we have learned how to harness the sun's energy. There is a real science to the way our brain and body have adapted to the solar world, so exploring the endocrinology of sunlight and darkness should be revealing.

There is a wealth of books and research articles written about the pineal gland, melatonin and melanin, so we can present the interrelationship between each topic in this chapter. Melanin was the sole topic in 1995 and melatonin and the pineal gland were discussed in 1996. In this chapter, we will explore the rhythmic connection that exists between the pineal gland, melatonin and our solar universe.

THE BLINDING OF THE THIRD EYE

To continue with the theme presented in the last chapter, our physical bodies are in constant communication with the surrounding universe. It is only natural that the human body has physiological functions that respond to and depend on the sun and other cosmic phenomena. There is a rhythm to life and our brain and body must keep up with this guiding force. Rhythm is one of the principles of the Kybalion and it pervades every life process. If we understand that man is a microcosm of the macrocosm (Principle of Correspondence), then it is simple to see how our bodies are intimately connected to nature. The major problem we encounter today is that we have detached ourselves from nature and we are out of tune. Our many work schedules, different diets, and unchallenging intellectual environments have led us away from nature's rhythm. We are actually out of tune with reality, and our third eye vision is blinded.

The pineal gland (or Third Eye) is a brain structure that has been studied since ancient times. Modern science has deemed the Greek anatomist Herophilos (325-280 B.C.) as the first one to discover the pineal gland as a "tap" or "sphincter" function for the ventricular system and the soul. In relief of the white-washed history textbooks that we are bombarded with in school, Dr. Richard King (1990) has provided us with an African-centered perspective on the history of the pineal gland. King (1990) has documented that the location of the pineal in the center of the head has been a site associated with spiritual illumination, and this discovery was not due to white scientists.

From an historical perspective, King informs us that Herophilos was actually interpreting knowledge stolen from Ancient African scientists who gave us the Egyptian Mystery System (see James, 1954). Upon viewing the unwrapping of King Tut's mummy, for example, there was found a golden bird that laid across the top of the crown of the head with outstretched wings covering the front of the head and the body of the bird along the center of the head. According to King, this may have been a symbolic statement that the location of the soul is in the brain's ventricular system because the shape of the bird closely resembles the top view appearance of the ventricular system. The lateral ventricles are similar to the outstretched wings and the bird's body is similar to the third and fourth ventricles (King, 1990).

In Chapter 2, it was stated that the shape of the melanocyte was the cellular KA (see Fig. 1). Although there are other divisions of the soul, KA and BA make up the first two divisions of the soul (Akbar, 1994). KA is the physical aspect of the soul that remains with the deceased and BA is the breath or spirit part of the soul that can leave the body. A human-headed bird, BA, was used by ancient

Africans to represent the soul. The Benu bird or stork was used to represent spirit. Thus, to find the symbolic soul-spirit bird placed atop King Tut's head at death and the many other representations of birds found on royal crowns throughout Egypt (or Kemet) represents the soul as an African concept. King provides solid evidence that the so-called discovery by Herophilos was already 1,000 years old in Africa.

The pineal derived its name through the efforts of Galenos (Galen of Pergamon, A.D. 130-200 A.D.). He considered the structure to be a "gland,'" separate from surrounding brain structures. In the human, the pineal has a "pine cone" shape so it was called *conarium*. The Latin word for pine cone was *pineale* (Binkley, 1988). In the 17th century, Rene Descartes (1596-1650) reinvigorated information from previous cultures and considered the pineal to be the "seat of the soul" (Descartes, 1649). The discovery of melatonin in the 20th century generated a new interest in the functioning of the pineal. According to King (1990), "inner vision, intuition, creative genius, and spiritual illumination were all found to be dependent upon the pineal gland blood born chemical messengers that controlled skin color and opened the hidden door to the darkness of the collective unconscious mind, allowing the ancient priest scientist to visualize knowledge from the mind's timeless collective unconscious memory banks."

From an evolutionary perspective, the morphological structure of the human anatomy may have changed over thousands of years. You can detect the obvious changes on the external surface of the body (e.g., skin color and hair), but the internal changes are less noticeable. Drastic fluctuations in the external environment can stimulate an internal change to allow humans to adapt to the conditions (e.g., higher metabolic rate in cold conditions). It is quite possible that structural change in the brain could occur over a long period of time by the way one cognitively processes information, and the way knowledge is obtained can have a significant impact on learning. The mental process of acquiring knowledge is a significant point because it has an influence on the way cultures are developed.

In finding a practical implication for her theory, Welsing (1991) informs us that the Color Confrontation thesis theorizes that the majority of the world's people, nonwhites, were manipulated into subordinate positions because, never having experienced such a state in terms of their own thought and logic processes and premises, they were unprepared to understand aggressive patterns of white behavior. Conversely, the constant invasion of foreigners to African dominated cultures (e.g., Ancient Kemet) stimulated an epistemological shift because the invaders could not comprehend the complex learning style they had never seen before. During this changing phase in history where Kemet changed from black to brown to white, there was a change in the way knowledge was obtained. The concepts associated with mental imagery radically changed and the use of hieroglyphics slowly faded (Moore, 1996). The pineal gland lost the ability to generate inner vision and function as a "third eye" in humans.

During ancient times, the scientists or priests developed the Mystery System of language and mathematical symbolism to simultaneously access the inner realms of consciousness and to preserve the ancient knowledge. According to James (1954), this system was used to conceal secret and mystical meaning of their doctrines from foreigners. Relative to our discussion, the amulet of the Eye of Horus is an example of a symbol that has deeper meaning (King, 1990). According to the myth, Heru fought his evil uncle Set to avenge the death of his father Osiris. In the battle, Heru's eye was torn to pieces, but with magic, Thoth, god of writing, assembled the pieces. The amulet was called "Sound Eye" because of its association with the regeneration of Heru's eye. The Eye of Heru is thus the third eye, a regenerated or transformed eye (King, 1990).

It is obvious that we are no longer able to think like both the ancient priests of Kemet and the scientists they learned from. In terms of losing the third eye inner vision of the pineal gland (Alder, 1968), the spiritual abilities may have closed when the procreative organs below opened (Percival, 1974) in the genital area. There really is no physiological purpose for a genital orgasm, so the orgasmic experience may be a vestigial consequence resulting from the opening of the procreative organs. Moreover, a genital orgasm may be a psychological reward to ensure humans will engage in copulation for its main purpose, reproduction. It is known that meditation can raise a force called Kundalini from the base of the spine to the top of the head and lead to an "awakening" or spiritual awareness (Greenwell, 1990). Those who are able to experience this mental tingling in the top of the head have reobtained the first orgasm the body has ever known.

Structurally, the human pineal gland is physically attached to the brain but it floats in cerebrospinal fluid in a cavity known as the fourth ventricle. The location is virtually in the center of the head and it is the source of the metaphysical "halo" seen around the head of those who have experienced spiritual enlightenment (e.g, Jesus, Buddha). It is possible that vibrations from the meditative experience could generate stimulation in the pineal gland and cause it move or become erect. Therefore, pineal stimulation may be synonymous with the erections experienced in the male penis and/or female clitoris. Due to changing thought patterns over thousands of years, erections are now experienced more so in the genitalia versus the inner organs in the brain, the pineal and the pituitary gland.

With the closing of these inner organs (i.e., pineal and pituitary), the eyes became blind to all but human physical things (Percival, 1974) and the ideas of others. The introduction of television and radio into our society has decreased our abilities to meditate and tune into self. As presented by Pookrum (1993), television and radio waves are sources of light. People who are mentally weak and unable to tune into the spiritual realm are controlled by base desires (e.g., lust, sex, money, material items and instant gratification) that can be manipulated via television and radio. Light no longer stimulated the pineal gland for inner vision, but it went through the sexual organ and was lost in nature. Releasing physical energy from having too much sex and always thinking about it can negatively affect a person's consciousness, reduce their level of awareness and drain their spiritual abilities. Furthermore, focusing on topics related to sex is an effective way to create mental diversion, to control behavior and to keep people passive and uninformed.

If you closely examine the exploitation of sex-related topics, then it is easy to see how sex can be used in modern society to sell material items and to manipulate minds in a calculated manner. Contemporary history reveals that a monopoly of powerful people have used sex as an effective tactic to control the thinking of a whole society during very critical moments in history. In the 1990s, for example, sexploitation in the media to control the thinking of the masses of people can be recalled from the media circuses centered around Clarence Thomas and Anita Hill, O.J. Simpson and Nicole Simpson and Bill Clinton and Monica Lewinsky. Now that we have reached 2001, the "powers that be" have thrown Jesse Jackson into the sex game during a critical time in American history when he was prepared to lead the masses in a demonstration to protest the 2000 election process. Although nearly two years old when the story was revealed to the public, we now have Jesse Jackson and Karin Stanford. For those who want to control the way society functions, it was very timely to expose Jesse Jackson's sexual affair to the public to apparently silence him and simultaneously dupe the masses.

All of these issues were private matters, but think of the amount of media attention that was devoted to make these household topics of discussion. Reflect on any meaning or reason to focus so much attention on those sexploitation topics. What about the Savings and Loans Crisis and the illegal selling of Junk Bonds that still affect our pocket books and the country's deficit? What about the manipulated Gulf war that wasted millions of dollars seeing smart and dumb bombs explode? The innocent Iraqi people were devastated and Saddam Hussein is still in power. What about the energy crisis facing the U.S.A. Residents in California have no electricity and residents throughout the country are unable to pay skyrocketing gas bills. What about the election debacle that put the son (George Bush, Jr.) of an ex-CIA administrator and ex-president (George Bush, Sr.) into the White House due to confusion in the state where his brother (Jeb Bush) is the governor? Can we really believe that out of all the people in the U.S. only the Bush Family is brilliant enough to lead this government? A rhetorical question is what in the world are the masses of people thinking about - SEX?

It is safe to say that our thinking and the knowledge base we have today is obtained on a different mental plane than the ancients. Modern scientists still debate and speculate how the ancients knew complex mathematics and how they mapped the geography of the earth as well as the cosmos. The scientific principles used by the ancients to create civilizations, to build the pyramids and to construct other massive monuments are unmatched by what we can mentally conceptualize. Today, we are ridiculously dependent on computers to generate what the mind could have the capacity to do. It is safe to say that the development of ancient science is unparalled because it was done when there were no computers, space shuttles, tractors, cranes, bulldozers or gas-powered machinery. Besides the construction of massive monuments, the metaphysical and interplanetary connections are additional achievements that make our civilization appear light years behind the ancients. Our third eye vision has been blinded.

MELATONIN

Before we discuss the third eye in detail, we will first define the hormone of darkness (melatonin) that has reawakened an interest in the scientific exploration of the pineal gland. In 1958, Lerner, Case, Takahashi, Lee and Mori isolated the pineal factor responsible for the blanching of frogs and showed it be an indole. The substance was given its name because it lightens skin (mela) and it is derived from serotonin (tonin). Since these initial observations, the synthesis of melatonin has been characterized in the following manner: tryptophan to 5-hydroxytryptophan to serotonin to N-acetylserotonin to melatonin. Three key enzymes are involved in this biosynthetic pathway and the rate limiting enzyme for melatonin synthesis is N-acetyltransferase (NAT). NAT converts serotonin into melatonin.
Although it is mentioned here as a precursor molecule, serotonin is a very important neurotransmitter that is highly associated with mood

disorders. For example, the antidepressant prozac functions as a serotonin uptake inhibitor to increase serotonin functioning in depressed patients (Stark, Fuller and Wong, 1985). Serotonin is released during the day from the pineal and melatonin is released at night from the pineal, and both neurohormones function to influence mood (Moore, 1996). Any alteration in either substance can disturb a person's biological rhythm (e.g., jet lag).

There are two well established roles for melatonin in animals and one role indicates where the name is derived. First, melatonin can lighten the skin of invertebrate species (Lerner et al., 1958). Secondly, melatonin can seasonally inhibit reproduction in mammals (Wurtman and Axelrod, 1965) during fall and winter months. Current research has provided a wider view of its potential to influence other bodily functions. The role of melatonin in Alzheimer's disease, reproduction, cancer, neurological functions, kidney activity, changes in body fat, and antioxidant activities have been reviewed (Watson, 1999).

In general, melatonin is known to be an effective antioxidant that can provide a youthful appearance. It is being studied as a key to understanding many of the nutritional and metabolic changes associated with diseases of aging. Restoration of melatonin production lost with increasing age has been shown to modify the actions of aging on lipid production, lipid peroxidation, tissue antioxidants, and cell functions. In addition to regulating certain aspects of aging, melatonin plays important roles in AIDS and some cancers by modulating metabolism and antioxidant nutrient status (Watson, 1999). In sum, we can understand the interest from the general public to mass consume melatonin.

THE PINEAL GLAND

The location of the pineal is figuratively a single-eye in the middle of the head of some lower vertebrates and reptiles. In lizards, for example, the pineal may protrude from the forehead. The pineal is close enough to the surface of the forehead in chickens that it functions as a light sensitive organ like the two lateral eyes (Binkley, 1988).

In mammals, the pineal gland rests between the two cerebral hemispheres (see Fig. 3) and weighs about 100 milligrams in man and 1 mg in the rat (Wurtman, Axelrod and Kelly, 1968). One scheme for how external light can stimulate pineal functioning does not suffice to explain regulation of the pineal because of species variation. For the purpose of our discussion, Fig. 4 represents a scheme that has been used for the laboratory rat can be used as a standard. In the rat, the retina in the eyes contain the photoreceptors for acquiring light and dark information. Light information from the retina is conveyed to the hypothalamus by the retinohypothalamic tract. This pathway leads to the suprachiasmatic nucleus (SCN) in the hypothalamus. The fibers from the eyes to the SCN are distinct from the fibers in the optic nerves which proceed to the lateral geniculate nucleus and the visual cortex. From the SCN, fibers pass through the median forebrain bundle to the spinal cord and superior cervical ganglia in the sympathetic nervous system. In the final path to the pineal, the pineal parenchymal cells are innervated by sympathetic nerves containing the neurotransmitter, norepinephrine. Norepinephrine stimulates the pineal gland to release melatonin in a clock-like fashion.

The post-ganglionic sympathetic fibers innervating the pineal provide nocturnal activation of melatonin secretion via alpha and beta adrenergic cyclic AMP-dependent activation of NAT. In addition to norepinephrine, other neurotransmitters and their receptors have been localized to the pineals of several mammals (Ebadi and Govitrapong, 1986; Ebadi et al., 1989). Moreover, the observation that factors other than light can modulate peak melatonin secretion (Vivien-Roels et al., 1993) suggests the complex nature of pineal functioning. In a review of pineal gland neuropeptides over the last two decades (see Benson, 1999), specific antibodies to neuropeptides of known structure have been developed and applied in immunocytochemical studies of mammalian pineal glands. Although the function of these fifteen or more neuropeptides is unknown, they are postulated to modulate pinealocyte melatonin synthesis and release. Neuropeptide Y, opioid peptides, substance P, somatostatin, vasopressin and oxytocin are a few of the uncommonly known pineal gland neuropeptides (Benson, 1999).

In response to light, experimental studies with animals have confirmed the pineal gland's role as a photoreceptor, endocrine gland, light transducer, regulator of regulators and circadian or biological clock. Biological clocks are cellular components that possess timing ability in an organism. The pineal is a biological clock (not the only proposed clock) in some species because it is capable of self-sustained oscillations *in vitro*. The oscillations may be circadian rhythms which are biological cycles that continue to oscillate in constant conditions with periods close to 24 hours. Light-dark information is used to "set" the biological clock. The pineal clock appears to be important for measuring night-length and day-length. Each period may fluctuate, but the measurement of either defines the relationship since the two must add up to 24 hours. There is evidence that the pineal can function by itself as a clock or photoreceptive organ, but these capabilities are not found in rats and humans.

In the rat, circadian clock information for the pineal gland primarily comes from the SCN. Lesions of the eyes or pathway that leads to the SCN does not disturb the pineal rhythm. However, lesions of the SCN or pathways leading to the pineal abolish the pineal rhythm. Due to these experimental manipulations, the hypothesis that has been proposed is that the circadian rhythm originates in cells of the SCN, and it is in the SCN that the information from the clock is integrated with information from the eyes about the prevailing light conditions.

Modern scientists are once again realizing that the rising and setting of the sun and the cyclical relationship between the sun and the moon are critical for all living systems. The pineal no longer receives direct stimulation from the sun in humans, but the pineal gland is one of the components of our discussion on the endocrinology of sunlight and darkness. The critical role of the pineal may be as a timekeeper (Binkley, Riebman and Reilly, 1977) or regulator of many cyclical biological activities. Periodic secretion of melatonin primarily at night provides a means for the pineal to send time signals to other parts of the body.

An interesting note can be made about this periodic secretion and the male genitalia. It is well documented that melatonin levels are higher at night and they subside as the dawn approaches. Although speculative, it is possible that the accumulation of melatonin during the night may have an effect on the highly pigmented penis during the early morning hours. In most males, the penis is surprisingly darker than other parts of the human body. Speculation on the evolutionary significance of pigmentation of the genitalia has been problematic (Kittles, 1995), however, Kittles hypothesized that skin color is affected by the thickness of the skin. Since the epidermis around the penis is extremely thin, it favors considerable exposure of melanin in the melanocytes and keratinocytes, causing the area to appear dark.

Even though the penis is rarely exposed to direct sunlight, the fact that it is darker than other parts of the human anatomy suggests a potential role for melatonin. Therefore, it is hypothesized that circulating levels of melatonin in the blood can assist in stimulating penile erections in the early morning.

Another cyclical melatonin effect that is less speculative is its role in mood disorders. For example, when the melatonin cycle is disturbed due to a change in the external environment, a person might develop Seasonal Affective Disorder (S.A.D.) or Winter Depression. During the winter months, the sun does not shine as long as it does during other seasons. For individuals who are light sensitive, the shorter days can affect brain hormones like melatonin. The most effective cure for S.A.D. is light therapy (Rosenthal et al., 1984; Yoon, 1996), so this is key evidence that the sun is important for elevating mood.

SOLTRIOL

In a sense, the sun is like a drug that affects numerous regulatory pathways. One very important regulatory pathway stimulated by the sun is the biosynthesis of Vitamin D (or Soltriol).

Soltriol was introduced by Stumpf in 1988 to describe this sun-derived hormone, so we will adopt it for the purpose of this discussion. We will refer to Vitamin D as a steroid hormone because to call it a vitamin is a misnomer. Therefore, the sun is like a drug that can stimulate the production of steroid hormones such as soltriol. We commonly think of soltriol as the substance fortified in or added to milk because the medical establishment has realized the detrimental effects of what a lack of soltriol can cause (e.g., weak bones and teeth).

Soltriol is widely believed to be the "calcium homeostatic steroid hormone" that acts peripherally with calcitonin and parathyroid hormone to regulate calcium levels in blood and tissues. The effect on calcium, however, is only one role of soltriol. Another perspective is that soltriol can act as a comprehensive somatotrophic activator and modulator. The new concept proposes that the steroid hormone soltriol is the skin-derived endocrine messenger of sunlight, functioning to coordinate the life processes of an organism's internal milieu with conditions in our solar environment. Soltriol may be a significant hormone helping to optimize an organism's development, growth, and reproduction (Stumpf, 1988). There is no mystery as to why cod liver oil (a food source for soltriol) is so important during the winter months.

Furthermore, melatonin is one of the major pineal hormones that have been linked to mammalian reproduction. Suppression of gonadal activities in relation to the daily and seasonal dark-light cycles is generally believed to be the main action of melatonin. In humans, melatonin functioning has been linked to mood disorders such as Seasonal Affective Disorder. Since there are binding sites for melatonin in several places in the central nervous system, there is a much more complex role than the regulation of reproduction.

In relation to the sun, soltriol and melatonin are the respective endocrine hormones for sunlight and darkness. The effect of sunlight on soltriol formation is regulated in the skin by melanin content and distribution (Stumpf and Privette, 1989). The role of melanin in the regulation of soltriol production can be described based on observations that the "hormone of sunlight," soltriol, stimulates melanin production *in vitro* (Tomita, Fukushima and Tagami, 1986), and that the "hormone of darkness," melatonin, lightens melanocytes (Lerner, Case Takahashi, Lee and Mori, 1958). It is suggested that this dual regulation produces an interactive relationship between the two endocrine systems in which soltriol is complimentary to the effects of melatonin.

From autoradiographic studies, it has been demonstrated that there are wide distribution sites for soltriol and melatonin binding in the nervous system and endocrine glands. There are strong potential influences of soltriol and melatonin on neural activities in diverse components of the central nervous system with effects on motor, sensory, endocrine and autonomic systems. The presence of melanin in these key areas and the skin can significantly influence the functioning of these complimentary hormones.

As an intermediary substance, melanin uses the sun to generate soltriol and possibly other steroid hormones. Stumpf and Privette (1989) stated that soltriol, like other steroid hormones, has target sites in the brain and therefore can be expected to have organizational effects on the developing brain. Furthermore, soltriol can induce permanent changes as well as activational effects on the mature brain. Organizational effects may include entrainment of certain biorhythms, while activational effects may include heightened mood, increased alertness, extrasensory perception and other responses and functions yet to be determined. The presence of melanin can only enhance these effects and cause transitory functional alterations in both the brain and the body.

PINEAL GLAND CALCIFICATION

Interestingly, there is a connection between calcium accumulation and the pineal gland. For example, experimental evidence demonstrates that melatonin production declines with age. One possible mechanism that may attribute to the decline is calcification of the pineal gland. If the pineal gland calcifies or hardens during the aging process this may lead to a lower production of melatonin. Therefore, melatonin's effects diminish with age. In the middle and latter decades of life, melatonin may decrease the youthful appearance of the skin, lower energy and mood level, decrease sleep time and no longer properly regulate many cyclical biological events. The melatonin craze in the 1990s was a wild attempt to turn back the aging process. As we have emphasized throughout this volume, dark does matter.

Skin color is certainly a factor involved in the calcification process. Pineal calcification may be clinically important as a radiological midline marker for the detection of intracranial displacements and a physiological marker for the pineal's control on soltriol-mediated homeostasis of calcium. King, Locke, King, Miles and Thompson (1994) reviewed 1,622 cases of pineal gland calcification in African Americans and defined an overall pineal gland calcification (PGC) incidence of 15.2%. Males in the group, 933 in number, had a PGC incidence of 16.6%. Females in the group, 689 in number, had a PGC incidence of 13.4%. According to King and colleagues, almost all reports of PGC have reported incidence rates for Africans of 5% to 9%, Asians 9% to 25% and Europeans of 50% or greater.

It is quite obvious that melanin in and outside of the body deserves special attention. The darkness of melanin can essentially serve as a sink for the accumulation of toxic substances, free radicals and ions. In terms of pineal calcification, intrapineal melanin may function as a calcium sink (King et. al, 1994) and contribute to the calcification process. There is experimental evidence that the effects of pineal calcification are minimal because a calcified pineal gland can still release melatonin. However, if we understand the evolutionary history of humans, then we can begin to uncover how significant environmental fluctuations over thousands of years can lead to structural changes in our internal physiology (Moore, 1995, 1996). For further reading, Kittles (1995) has provided a thorough review of the nature, origin, and variation of human pigmentation to highlight the distinction we are attempting to make between darkly pigmented humans of African descent and less pigmented humans of European descent.

The incidence of pineal calcification and S.A.D. are higher in lighter pigmented people. The environmental conditions, however, can determine the severity of theses abnormalities. It does not mean that darkly pigmented people cannot develop these problems, but it is emphasized that a lack of and diminished output of sun-derived biological mechanisms (i.e., melanin, soltriol, pineal functioning and melatonin) can greatly reduce the quality of life both mentally and physically. Under ideal temperate conditions ranging between 65 to 80 degrees Fahrenheit, the endocrinology of sunlight and darkness can function with relative ease. Traveling to and living in the Tropics does a lot for your mental and physical health since the sun basically shines 365 days of the year.

On the other hand, the absence of these sun-derived biological mechanisms may be advantageous under certain cold, less lighted environmental conditions. For example, any animal or human living in a cold, sun-depleted environment must have physiological mechanisms to adapt to the harsh conditions. Dark skin pigmentation is no longer as important to block the harmful effects of solar radiation. Therefore, lighter skin is an adaptation. The pineal control of melatonin and soltriol are no longer as important due to a lack of stimula tion from the sun. Interestingly, one of the functions of melatonin is to retract melanin granules in melanocytes to allow more light to penetrate the skin. Melatonin can lighten the skin, but it is not needed when the sun is not a factor. Soltriol is generated by the sun, so calcium absorption from soltriol synthesis would be less important when the full force of the sun is reduced. Pineal calcification would be the end result of these harsh environmental changes. The brain and body would no longer be as responsive to the transitory functional alterations controlled by the pineal-melatonin-soltriol-melanin connection. Other functional alterations would become more imperative.

For example, living in the cold would require higher metabolic processes. Animal data (Vriend, 1983) has provided evidence for a link between the pineal gland modulation of the neuroendocrine-thyroid axis. The thyroid secretes thyroxine (T4) which is important for elevating body metabolism. More heat can be generated with a functioning thyroid gland. Therefore, living in the cold could be tolerated with the increase body metabolism.

Experiments with rats and hamsters have provided evidence for an inhibitory action of the pineal gland on the neuroendocrine-thyroid axis (Vriend, 1983). According to the experimental manipulations, endogenous melatonin could account for the inhibitory action of the pineal gland on blood T4 levels. In other words, decreased melatonin during cold, sun-depleted environmental conditons can actually increase thyroid activity. Furthermore, the effects of melatonin on the neuroendocrine-thyroid axis are similar to its effects on the neuroendocrine-gonadal axis.

Melatonin suppression of the neuroendocrine-thyroid axis and the neuroendocrine-gonadal axis suggests a common site of action for the thyroid and gonadal effects. Therefore, it is quite possible that evolutionary descendants of people from Europe have an overall lower secretion of melatonin and a lower reproductive rate due to a malfunctioning pineal gland.

In conclusion, our physical connection to the universe is through the nervous system. The brain contains the necessary organs to keep us in rhythm with the cosmos, and the pineal gland and melatonin have a contributory role in the endocrinology of sunlight and darkness. The sun-derived hormone soltriol is also a critical factor that helps to establish and maintain positive physical and mental health.

Next, we will discuss melanin in the brain (i.e., neuromelanin). Similar to the dark surface of the penis which receives no direct sunlight, there are dark areas in the brain which do not receive sunlight. These dark brain regions correlate with the presence of catecholamines. Neuromelanin is not secreted like catecholamines, however, and it does not respond to sunlight and darkness. The only endocrinology connection with neuromelanin is the fact that neuromelanin can absorb neurotransmitters and affect their release pattern. As we will explore in the next chapter, neuromelanin is also important for the proper maintenance of physical and mental health.

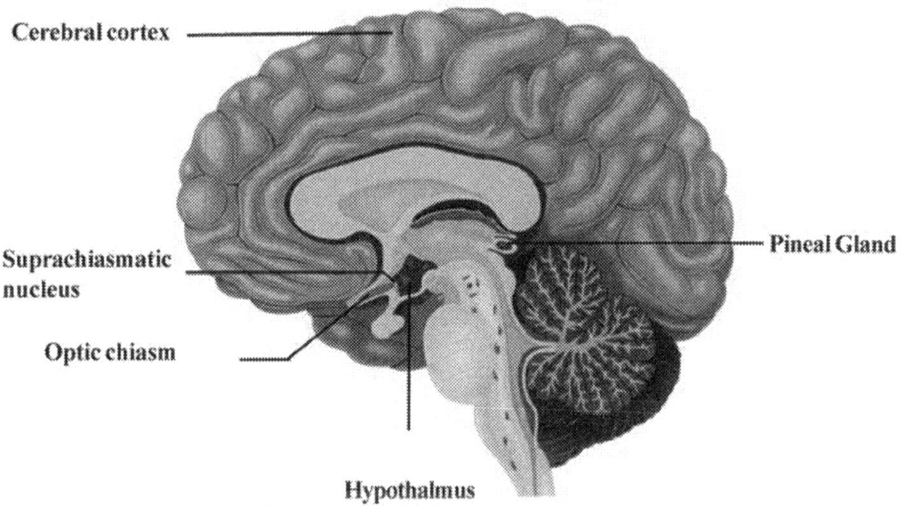

Figure 3 - A sagittal section of the human brain illustrating the relative location of twelve cell groups (black dots) containing neuromelanin in the brainstem and the midbrain. The pineal gland is located in the upper portion of these pigmented neurons.

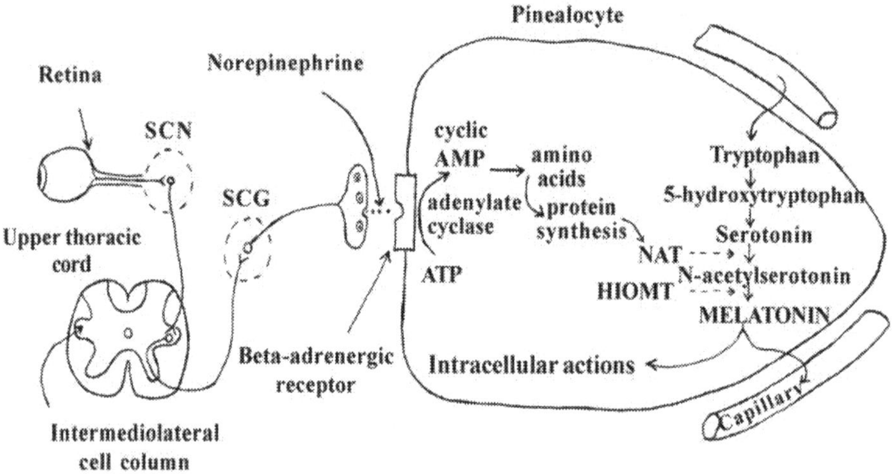

Figure 4 - Neural Pathway from the eye to the pineal gland and the synthesis of pineal hormones. The pathway extends from the eye to the suprachiasmatic nucleus (SCN) in the hypothalamus to the spinal cord to the superior cervical ganglia (SCG) and then innervates the pineal gland. A beta-adrenergic receptor is activated and chemical events occur to produce melatonin.

Chapter 5

Dark Matter in the Brain

The scientific term used to describe dark matter in the brain is neuromelanin. It is different in structure than the melanin found in the skin; however, it is commonly called neuromelanin because it is pigmented tissue located deep within the brain. Obviously, the pigmented tissue in the brain is neither a direct nor an indirect effect from the sun. Since the sun does not darken brain tissue, nature must have provided a reason for the presence of dark matter in the brain. It sounds as though neuromelanin is cloaked in mystery, but its presence in the brain cannot be denied. In this chapter, we will review scientific research that provides clues to why neuromelanin may exist.

BACKGROUND INFORMATION

Multidisciplinary investigations from fields such as molecular biology, biochemistry and neuroscience have helped to advance our understanding of dark matter in the brain. The advantages of melanin functioning have already been discussed (Moore, 1995), but this does not negate the fact that new explorations are being conducted daily in research laboratories throughout the world. Experiments from places such as the U.S.A., Japan and Europe are shedding light on our understanding of neuromelanin. In general, neuromelanin can function as a neutralizer of harmful toxic substances, a nerve conduction facilitator and an energy transformer. All three functions highlight the importance of having melanin in the brain.

Despite the advancements that have been made in melanin research, the structure and specific role of neuromelanin remain difficult to scientifically analyze. Neuromelanin is a granular, dark pigment that may range from brown to black. It is not found in every part of the brain, but it is located in areas where neurotransmitters like dopamine and norepinephrine are synthesized. It is confirmed that neuromelanin occurs almost exclusively in catecholaminergic neurons, which are involved in conscious perception, movement, emotion and memory (Bogerts, 1981). Dark does matter in certain areas of the brain and neuromelanin may provide a link to higher states of consciousness (Barr, 1983).

The biosynthesis of neuromelanin is a point of controversy. The highest levels of neuromelanin are found in the neurons of the substantia nigra and locus coeruleus, which are known to contain relatively high concentrations of dopamine and norepinephrine, respectively (Prota, 1992). The question, however, is how does neuromelanin form? In the skin, tyrosinase is a key enzyme leading to melanin formation. However, there has been no positive confirmation that tyrosinase is in pigmented brain tissue (Rodgers and Curzon, 1975). The normal pigmentation of the substantia nigra in human albinos (Foley and Baxter, 1958), who lack all peripheral tyrosinase, is also consistent with tyrosinase not being involved in neuromelanin formation.

The connection to catecholamine biosynthesis cannot be overlooked. The apparent association of neuromelanin with catecholamine production in the brain is generally regarded as indirect proof of the involvement of dopamine and related metabolites in the biosynthesis of the pigment (Barnes, 1988). Other than the precursor enzymes (e.g., phenylalanase or tyrosine hydroxylase), which convert amino acids to make catecholamines, the degradative enzyme monoamine oxidase (MAO) may appear to affect neuromelanogenesis. MAO can breakdown catecholamines and terminate their neurochemical activity. Prota (1992) reviewed evidence that MAO, coupled with nonenzymatic oxidative processes, is mainly responsible for neuromelanin formation. The MAO connection is still speculative, but it supports data from earlier years. Another hypothesis that has received less attention is the possibility that neuromelanin is capable of self-synthesis (Barr, 1983).

In Barr's massive review on melanin, a highly significant point was made that the functions of neuromelanin are due to a "change in state" rather than a change in concentration. Therefore, it is not so much the quantity of melanin in the brain but the quality of its content or physical condition. If neuromelanin is an organizing molecule capable of self-synthesis, then its presence can be genetically determined to function differently depending upon the animal species or the ethnic origin of the human.

Although lower animals are used to study the function of the nervous system and to define human behavior, there are multiple behavioral phenomena that highlight the inadequacy of some animal models. Humans are specially constructed to have a thinking capacity that far exceeds the mental, spiritual (if any) and physical abilities of lower animals. Having dark matter can provide an even greater enhancement of "hueman" possibility. The absence of color, even in the animal world, is considered a genetic abnormality. In general, the amount of neuromelanin in the brain varies in the different animal species, being greatest in man and progressively lower as the relation to man becomes lower (Marsden, 1983). Laboratory animals such as rats, mice, guinea pigs and rabbits have little or no neuromelanin. According to the varied sources of experimental data, it is suggested that brain melanin is genetically programmed to function at different capacities depending upon a person's overall genetic capacity to produce melanin (Moore, 1995).

NERVE CONDUCTION FACILITATOR

In heavily pigmented neurons, neuromelanin granules are closely packed, dispersed through the cytoplasm, and extend into the axon hillock and initial portions of the axon. Neuromelanin is less abundant in the dendrites and is absent in the neuronal processes remote from the cell bodies. In other words, a microscopic analysis of a single brain cell or neuron reveals that neuromelanin does not saturate every component of the neuron. It is primarily located in the cytoplasm where neurotransmitters are synthesized and where a host of other cellular activities occur. The axon hillock is a site where a nerve impulse is generated to be sent down the axon, so the presence of melanin in the axon hillock suggests a role in neurotransmission.

Neuromelanin does not extend down the entire axon and it is less detected in the dendritic portions of the neuron. Since it is absent from the dendrite, it appears to be less involved with receiving information and more involved with generating nerve impulses.

McGinness, Cory and Proctor (1974) performed some laboratory investigations on the electronic properties of melanin to reveal that the nervous system utilizes certain voltages, and that this electrical energy is harnessed by melanin. The authors stated that the threshold switching at low gradients poses some theoretical questions. In effect, there is more activity elicited from melinated brain regions when compared to non-melinated brain regions.

It is suggested that the bioelectronic properties associated with melanin can help to facilitate nerve conduction in the following three ways: 1) it can speed the pace of nerve impulses; 2) it can concentrate ions for high voltage generating activity; and 3) it can provide an electrochemical surge.

The first point indicates that melanin can help to transfer specific chemical molecules, and subsequently, speed the nerve impulses in highly melinated brain regions. Since melanin can act as an electron-transfer agent, it can cause the nerve cell to exhibit more activity by facilitating the electrical and chemical transmission of nerve impulses.

The second point relates directly to the accumulation of electrolytes or charged ions in melinated brain regions. The more charges in a cell can translate into a higher voltage in the cell. Therefore, melinated brain regions can aggregate charged ions and produce high voltage generating activity. As a result, the high voltage generating activity could have a facilitative effect on the nerve impulse.

The third point suggest that melanin can cause a greater release of neurochemicals from nerve cells. Neural transmission requires the stimulation of certain ions or electrolytes across the cell membrane. As a result of this change in the cell membrane, neurochemicals are released from the cell to transmit a nerve impulse. Interestingly, there are several brain regions (e.g., substantia nigra, locus coeruleus, raphe nucleus) that have both high melanin content and neurochemical activity (e.g., dopamine, norepinephrine, serotonin). Therefore, melanin can increase the voltage, cause an electrochemical surge, and positively influence the release of neurochemicals.

It was first suggested by McGinness in 1972 that melanin may act as an amorphous semiconductor, that is a threshold switch. McGinness theorized about the electronic properties of melanin reported by Blois (1969, 1971), who observed a rise in the conductivity of melanin under an applied voltage. McGinness suggested that this rise might be a result of increased kinetic energy of the electrons leading to higher mobility and promotion to excited states. In other words, melanin may act as a threshold switch to "pump up the volume" from a lower voltage to a higher voltage.

In sum, the bioelectronic properties of melanin facilitate nerve conduction and generate much more activity than non-melinated brain regions. It is very critical that melanin is found in the nervous system because it helps to heighten mental awareness, it speeds up reaction time, and it greatly enhances the capacity of the brain to transmit nerve impulses. Consequently, the special properties associated with melanin in the nervous system can help to increase survival of the organism.

ENERGY TRANSFORMER

The consistent appearance of melanin in living organisms at locations where energy conversion or charge transfer occurs (skin, retina, midbrain, and inner ear) is of particular interest. Melanin is strategically placed in these locations to absorb and convert various forms of electromagnetic energy into energy states that can be used by the nervous system. Melanin is found in the skin to absorb ultraviolet light, in the retina to increase visual acuity and reaction time, in the midbrain to perform complex motor tasks, and in the inner ear to amplify sound. In all of these instances, melanin may be acting as an electronic device (McGinness et al.,1974).

The fact that melanin is black or dark in color could explain how it is functioning as a converter of energy. Since dark skin or any black substance absorbs heat, light is not reradiated, but it is converted to rotational and vibrational degrees of freedom (McGinness and Proctor, 1973). Contrary to blackness, whiteness reflects light. As a result pigmented cells are more capable of converting energy versus non-pigmented cells. Although there are comparable distributions of neuromelanin in the brain, darker colored people have a more modified external pigmentary system that has a greater capacity for charge transfer.

There are other physical mechanisms by which melanin can influence electrical energy. It has been proposed (Lacy, 1984: McGinness et al., 1973) that phonon-electron coupling is the possible transducing mechanism in bioelectronic processes involving neuromelanin. In other words, melanin is involved in the transformation of one form of energy into another by coupling together two different physical states (vibrations and electricity). The black appearance of melanin suggests that the phonon-electron coupling in this material may be particularly efficient for transforming energy. In the case of sunlight, the absorbed radiation is retained and transferred to excited electronic states. This excited physical state can explain the pleasant mood one may have on a bright, sunny day.

NEUTRALIZER OF TOXIC SUBSTANCES

Melanin is effective as a device for radiation-less conversion of the energy of harmfully excited molecules into innocuous vibrational energy (McGinness and Proctor, 1973). This conversion may deactivate metabolically excited molecules that can become potentially damaging to cells. Since there are no mechanical devices involved, that is why this conversion is called radiation-less. The important point is that melanin helps to ensure that the spread of further cellular damage is neutralized.

Melanin is also known to protect against dangerous free radicals. Free radicals are highly reactive chemical species that have an odd number of electrons, and hence, one unpaired electron. It has been proposed (Commoner, Townsend and Pake, 1954) that melanin acts like a deposit site for unpaired electrons, thus removing reactive free radicals. Peroxides are examples of chemical substances that can lose an electron and change into dangerous and cytotoxic substances.

The stable nature of melanin also gives it the unique feature to accumulate several biological compounds. For example, various amines, drugs, and a number of metals can be retained in melinated regions of the body for a very long time (Larsson and Tjalve, 1979). Lindquist, Larsson and Lyden-Sokolowski (1987) suggested that melanin's capacity to accumulate and bind a variety of compounds can allow neuromelanin to protect the cells that harbor the pigment by keeping potentially harmful substances bound, and thereafter, slowly releasing the agents in low, non-toxic concentrations.

What this means is that the level of melanin in the human body can significantly influence potential drug effects. As expressed by Barnes (1988), the slow release may cause certain drugs (e.g., cocaine) to have greater potency in highly melinated individuals, and subsequently, increase the rate of drug addiction in the Black community. When the skin is exposed to these biological substances, the damage can be observed by inspecting the skin. Within the brain, however, it is only possible during post-mortem studies to visualize the cellular changes caused by cytotoxicity. The brain is more delicate and complex than most other organs in the body. If the brain is saturated and overburdened with these cytotoxic molecules, then behavior is ultimately disturbed.

NEUROMELANIN PATHOLOGY

In terms of behavior, loss of pigment in the brain is more detrimental than loss of pigment in the skin. It has been well known for some years that in systemic tissues melanin is a double-edged sword. On the one hand it can act as an antioxidant, but in the presence of transitional metals (iron, manganese), solvents (carbon sulfide), poisonous gas (carbon monoxide) and certain drugs (meperidine, methamphetamine), it promotes the formation of reactive oxygen free radicals (Youdim, Ben-Shachar and Reiderer, 1994). We will present some pathologies associated with neuromelanin dysfunctioning and begin with Parkinson's Disease, the most common neuropathology.

Parkinson's Disease

Parkinson's Disease (PD) is a distinct clinical and neuropathological disease. It is clinically characterized by slow movements, resting tremor, muscle rigidity, and postural reflex impairment and pathologically by the loss of pigmented neurons, most prominently in the substantia nigra (SN). It is commonly believed that Lewy bodies, eosinophilic cytoplasmic inclusions, are the cellular marker for PD pathology (Marsden, 1983, Tanner, 1992).

Approximately one million Americans have this neurological disorder and more than 50,000 new patients are diagnosed each year. The problems can begin with a lack of facial expression, slowness of movement and weak voice. There may be a gradual increase in more noticeable problems such as shuffling steps, muscle stiffness and problems with balance. Eventually, the PD patient may experience severe immobility and intellectual decline.

The potential causes for these devastating effects have been scientifically investigated for over 100 years. Although PD has been researched for more than a century, the cause of the degeneration of dopamine-containing cells in the SN in PD patients is unknown. The different ways in which neuromelanin or its precursors might be toxic to pigmented nerve cells obviously invites speculation on its role in the cause of PD. One concept that has been used pertains to oxidative stress.

According to this concept, oxidative stress might be caused by either the actions of a neurotoxin or through the altered metabolism of dopamine (Jenner, 1992). Oxidative stress can cause dopamine cell death due to excessive formation of oxygen radical species (McGreer et al., 1989), and the altered dopamine metabolism may produce toxic species and indirectly implicate neuromelanin.

The autoxidation of dopamine to neuromelanin proceeds via semiquinone intermediates, which might be toxic to dopamine cells (Graham, 1978). The metabolism and breakdown of dopamine by MAO produces hydrogen peroxide, which may then be transformed into more toxic hydroxyl radicals, a process catalyzed by the presence of iron (Cohen, 1987). One suggestion is that dopamine metabolism is altered in the early stages of the disease such that there is increased dopamine synthesis and turnover and that this in turn leads to the excessive production of hydroxyl radicals and an acceleration of the rate of decay of dopamine neurons (Jenner, 1992).

The decay was thought to create the "waste product" called neuromelanin. Since neuromelanin in individual neurons from human SN or locus coeruleus increase sevenfold from the first decade in life to the eighth decade in life (Mann and Yates, 1974; Graham, 1979), it was postulated that catecholamine neurons may degenerate over time and form neuromelanin as the result of life-long injury from the by-products of catecholamine oxidation.

Auto-oxidation of catecholamines, by which is meant their non-enzymic oxidation by molecular oxygen, results in the univalent reduction of oxygen. As a consequence, hydrogen peroxide and superoxide radicals are formed, which may interact to produce the highly reactive hydroxyl radical and singlet oxygen within cells. To prevent these free radicals from causing cellular destruction, principal enzymes such as superoxide dismutase, catalase, and glutathione peroxidase are present to protect against oxygen-radical reactions in human cells (Marsden, 1983). As stated earlier in this chapter, the enzyme MAO may also be involved in neuromelanogenesis. MAO-B plays an important role in the induction of oxidative stress, and the normal increase in the activity of MAO-B with age may potentiate free radical formation (Danielczyk et al., 1988, Humfrey et al., 1990; Young and Perry, 1986).

Other than oxidative stress, there has been speculation about a potential toxin that selectively destroys dopamine-containing cells in the SN. One likely candidate is MPTP, a compound produced during illicit synthesis of a narcotic related to meperidine (Langston et al.,

1983). MPTP toxicity was discovered after inadvertent self-administration by drug abusers. Investigations of the mechanisms of MPTP toxicity have produced insights regarding the possible pathogenesis of PD because the users rapidly developed a movement disorder that closely resembled PD. MPTP-induced Parkinsonism is remarkable in that it strictly mimics the anatomic and clinical features of PD rather than causing more widespread CNS injury.

The mechanism of action of MPTP involves its metabolism by MAO-B to produce MPDP, which in turn is converted to the toxic agent, MPP+, that causes the cellular death. The toxic oxidation product reaches the extracellular fluid and then is transported by the dopamine transporter into dopamine terminals. Inhibition of MAO-B or the dopamine transporter protects against MPTP-generated MPP+ toxicity. MPTP is not a normal constituent of the environment and, therefore, cannot be responsible for more than a few cases of PD. Nevertheless, MPTP remains the "best" model for investigating PD to date. In addition, neurotoxins such as 6-hydroxydopamine (6-OH-DA), iron, and methamphetamine have been implicated. At present no lead compound has emerged as a candidate for the cause of PD.

Other than toxicant exposure, epidemiological studies have included age, gender, race, genetic predisposition, infection, trauma and emotional stress as other risk factors for PD (Tanner 1992). Of these many risk factors, "race" is related to the main topic of our discussion. Epidemiological reports still use this sociological construct called race to categorize people, but the emphasis should be placed on ethnicity. At least 20 studies over the last three decades were reviewed by Tanner (1992) and the highest rates of PD were in Europe and North America, whereas rates in Japan, China and Africa are markedly lower. These data have been interpreted to indicate a greater risk for PD among whites. It was stated earlier that brain melanin is genetically programmed to function at different capacities depending upon a person's overall genetic capacity to produce melanin. Numerous community-based epidemiologic studies throughout various regions of the world support this postulation that ethnicity can have a significant influence on melanin functioning.

In a Parsi community of Bombay, India, prevalence was similar to that found in Europe and North America. The Parsi are relatively recent immigrants to India and form a closed community into which conversion is impossible. This led Tanner (1992) to conclude that, "Although socioeconomic or environmental factors may explain the prevalence differences cited here, a still to be refuted possibility is that PD is more common in whites, most likely as a result of a common genetic characteristic." The conclusion from both epidemiologic and metabolic studies is that a combination of environmental factors plus genetic susceptibility to toxic action are responsible for PD than either of these factors alone (Jenner, 1992).

Other Neurodegenerative Disorders

In addition to PD, it is possible that neuromelanin may contribute to other neurodegenerative disorders such as multiple sclerosis, schizophrenia, neuroleptic malignant syndrome and idiopathic torsion dystonia. These neurodegenerative disorders have a different biogenetic origin, but they all may involve neuromelanin as a common link. There are specific genetic mutations that attribute to the manifestation of each disorder to suggest an inherited susceptibility to the disease. People of African descent are less likely to develop these abnormalities, so there may be a genetic advantage to thwart off these brain disorders.

In 1996, scientists from the National Institutes of Health identified a genetic link for PD from the DNA of patients (Polymeropoulos et al., 1996). The impact of their finding indicates that a single gene alteration somewhere within a region of DNA on the long arm of chromosome 4 can cause the disease. The researchers identified the gene region by studying the DNA of 28 members of a large Italian family containing almost 600 people. People in this family, some of whom migrated to the United States between 1890 and 1920, can trace their ancestry to a single couple who lived in Italy in the 18th century. More than 60 family members on both sides of the Atlantic have been diagnosed with PD.

Another Parkinson's-like disorder, Wilhelsen-Lynch disease (disinhibition-dementia-parkinsonian-amyotrophy complex), has been linked to a region of chromosome 17. A defect in mitochondrial DNA, which is separate from a person's chromosomes, has been linked to sporadic PD with unusual symptoms. Other genetic mutations may also play a role in some cases.

Multiple sclerosis is a CNS demyelinating disease that may have a genetic link to melanin functioning (Contantinescu, 1995). Significant evidence supports an autoimmune mechanism in the development of multiple sclerosis, activated by putative environmental factors in genetically predisposed individuals. Genetic factors strongly influence the susceptibility to demyelinating diseases in humans and rodents. Understanding the mechanisms governing susceptibility versus resistance may help to identify individuals at risk or design therapeutic strategies. Constantinescu (1995) formulated an hypothesis that resistance to multiple sclerosis is associated with dark skin pigmentation. While melanin may have a protective role against environmental factors which produce oxidative damage, the mechanism postulated here is that susceptibility to autoimmune demyelination is influenced by hormonal factors. The neurohormones melatonin and melanocyte stimulating hormone, which have opposing effects on immune functions, are simultaneously important determinants of the individual's production of melanin.

Geneticists have attempted to explain almost all aspects of human existence, from human evolution to food preferences and personality quirks. But one thing they have a hard time explaining is the persistence of certain disease genes over time. After all, if one is to believe the theory of natural selection, harmful mutations should be eliminated from human populations, not retained. Yet not only are certain harmful mutations not eliminated, some actually become more prevalent. For example, the gene causing a debilitating movement disorder called idiopathic torsion dystonia (ITD) has dramatically risen in a select community of Europeans (Hoffman, 1995).

The prevalence of the mutant ITD gene has risen dramatically over the past 350 years in Ashkenazi Jews - those of eastern

European extraction. ITD is characterized by abnormal movements and postures (Inzelberg, Flash, Schechtman and Korczyn, 1995). The exact anatomical site affected in ITD is unclear, but data points to the putamen, caudate, or thalamus as the major affected structures. Essentially, ITD is another movement disorder that may result from a lack of melanin functioning. A lack of the overall ability to produce melanin appears to make humans more susceptible to neurodegenerative disorders.

Schizophrenia, another neurodegenerative disorder, will be presented here to conclude this section on neuromelanin pathology. Hypopigmentation of SN does not seem to be a general finding in schizophrenia (Kaiya, 1980). However, low melanin content of SN may be a risk factor for catatonic syndromes, which can be elicited by neuroleptic treatment. An interesting case study about a 19 year old white German has shed light on the impact of low melanin content in the SN and the development of neuroleptic malignant syndrome (NMS) (Gertz and Schmidt, 1991). NMS is a rare, but life-threatening complication of neuroleptic treatment. Its symptoms are rigidity, fever, and autonomic dysfunction. It is typically associated with high potency neuroleptics when used in larger doses or when there is a rapid increase in total daily drug dose (Caroff, 1980; Shalev and Munitz, 1986).

According to Gertz and Schmidt (1991), the patient was brought to a psychiatric city hospital because he had expressed feelings of guilt and persecution, had become increasingly lethargic, sleepless, and developed incoherence in speech. There was no family history of mental illness; or had he any history of abnormalities during his development or any evidence of drug abuse. A preliminary diagnosis of a first episode of schizophrenia was made, and the patient was treated initially with haloperidol and levomepromazine. After five weeks of neuroleptic treatment, he died of an unknown cause.

Histological examination of the brain revealed a low melanin content in neurons in the SN. Since neuromelanin in the SN is thought to be the end product of non-enzymatic dopamine degradation, the amount of melanin probably depends on the overall amount of dopamine produced during life. Thus, dopamine production must have been low in the reported case.

Other than this one NMS clinical case, oxidative stress in melinated cells from substances such as iron and prostaglandins may potentially cause schizophrenia. In one study, iron bound to neuromelanin in melanized dopamine neurons was detected only in parkinsonian brains and not in controls (Ben-Shachar and Youdim, 1993). The interaction of iron with neuromelanin as identified by x-ray defraction technique was identical to iron interaction with synthetic dopamine melanin. In the absence of an identified exogenous or endogenous neurotoxin in idiopathic PD, iron-melanin interaction in the SN may serve as a candidate for the oxygen-radical induced neurodegeneration of the melanin containing dopaminergic neurons.

Binding of iron and metal ions to neuromelanin and its oxidative cytotoxicity in the pathogenesis of neurodegenerative disorders has been extensively studied (Enoch et al., 1994; Zecca et al., 1994, 1996; Faraldi et al., 1994; Shima et al., 1997; Aime et al., 1996). In general, the overload of neuromelanin is neurotoxic. Other toxic reactions can occur with prostaglandin in the brain.

Smythies (1996;1997) has made the connection between prostaglandin synthesis and the pathogenesis of schizophrenia. The presence of prostaglandins in the brain are not usually associated with brain injury. Damage in the periphery where a flesh wound (e.g., cut) may appear on the surface of the body is where prostaglandins commonly exert their effects. However, it is hypothesized that neuromelanin toxicity may stimulate the production of prostaglandins in the brain. Prostaglandin E2 , a cyclo-oxygenase metabolite of arachidonic acid, is released from damaged cells and produces hyperalgesia and sensitizes nociceptors (i.e., receptors for pain). The reason why aspirin and other nonsteroidal anti-inflammatory analgesics are effective in controlling pain is because they inhibit the cyclo-oxygenase enzyme, preventing the synthesis of prostaglandin.

Smythies (1996) hypothesized that one of the functions of neuromelanin in catecholamine neurons in the brain is to protect the cell against toxic quinones (such as dopaminochrome and noradrenochrome, or their dihydroxy isomers). Toxic quinones are produced from the catecholamines dopamine and noradrenaline (and possibly adrenaline) during the course of prostaglandin synthesis by the enzyme prostaglandin H synthase, or possibly by spontaneous oxidation. According to Smythies, there are aminochrome or adrenochromes that have been shown to be neurotoxic and to have psychomimetic properties in humans. In sum, the site of production of these compounds may be involved in the pathogenesis of PD or schizophrenia.

NEUROMELANIN PROTECTION

Protecting yourself from neuromelanin toxicity is possible because there are millions of elderly people who never succumb to the devastating disorders mentioned in this section. The inheritance of genes that lead to the production of high levels of melanin (internal as well as external) is the most adequate way to slow the production of toxicity in the brain. We ingest numerous pesticides, metal ions and industrial toxins from our diet and from the air we breathe. The greater the concentration of these potentially toxic agents in your immediate surroundings can increase your susceptibility to neuromelanin toxicity. It is important to be aware of the chemicals you are exposed to and the foods you digest because the protective role of neuromelanin against toxic substances can actually be detrimental to behavioral functioning. If neuromelanin is acting as a sink for harmful free radicals and/or toxic substances, it will eventually develop into a neurotoxic sponge.

Melanin and melatonin are scientifically known to be effective antioxidants produced by the body. When compared by age, people with melinated skin look younger than their age-matched melanin deficient counterpart. Antioxidants protect the body from toxic agents that can destroy cells and hasten the aging process. Not everyone has a melanin rich internal and external milieu, so enhancement with antioxidants may be effective. One of the reasons for the wild frenzy to mass consume melatonin in the 1990s was for its antioxidant properties.

Internal mechanisms to thwart neuromelanin pathology are difficult to assess. However, evidence from dietary intake of factors that interfere with the pathogenetic mechanism underlying PD have provided insight on how to prevent disease development (Tanner, 1992). For example, if oxidative mechanisms are involved in the pathogenesis of PD, intake of antioxidant vitamins may be protective (Cross et al., 1987). Consumption of foods rich in tocopherol (Vitamin E) decreased the risk of developing PD in two case-control studies, one comparing patients to spouses (Golbe, Cody and Duvoisin, 1986; Golbe et al., 1990). The use of supplemental multivitamins, vitamin E, or cod liver oil was similarly associated with a decreased risk for PD (Tanner, Cohen, Summerville and Goetz, 1988). Other than the sun, cod liver oil is a natural source of soltriol and this presents a more important role for the aforementioned endocrinology of sunlight (soltriol) and darkness (melatonin).

In sum, eating foods rich in tocopherol, soltriol or some other associated dietary factors may prevent the pathogenesis of neuromelanin. When investigating epidemiological studies, areas with a low prevalence of PD may not be those with a lesser concentration of environmental toxins but rather those in which there is higher dietary intake of protective substances (Tanner, 1992).

REFERENCES

Adams, J.D. and Odunze, I.N. (1991). Oxygen free radicals and Parkinson's disease. Free Radical Biological Medicine, 10, 161-169.

Akbar, N. (1994). Light from Ancient Africa. Tallahassee, FL: Mind Productions & Associates, Inc.

Alder, V.S. (1968). The Finding of the Third Eye. Maine: Samuel Weiser, Inc. Originally published 1938.

Amen, N.A. (1993). The Ankh: African Origin of Electromagnetism. Jamaica, NY: Nur Ankh Amen Press.

Aime, S., Fasano, M., Bergamasco, B., Lopiano, L. and Quattrocolo, G. (1996). Nuclear magnetic resonance spectroscopy characterization and iron content determination of human mesecephalic neuromelanin. Advances in Neurology, 73(69), 263-270.

Andrews, M. (1989). Color Me Right...Then Frame Me in Motion. Tennessee: Seymour-Smith Inc.

Bagnara, J.T. and Hadley, M.E. (1973). Chromatophores and Color Change. Englewood Cliffs, NJ: Prentice Hall.

Barnes, C. (1988). Melanin: The Chemical Key to Black Greatness,Vol.1. Houston, Texas: C.B. Publishers.

Barnes, C. (1993). Jazzy Melanin: A Novel. Houston, Texas: Melanin Technologies.

Barr, F.E. (1983). Melanin: the organizing molecule. Medical Hypothesis, 11(1), 1-140.

Barrenas, M.L. and Lingren, F. (1990). The influence of inner ear melanin on susceptibility to TTS in humans. Scanda. Audiol., 19, 97-102.

Beamoun, A. and Hughes, J. (1979). Biology of opioid peptides. Annual Review in Pharmacological Toxicology, 19, 245-267.

Ben-Shachar, D. and Youdim, M.B.H. (1993). Iron, melanin and dopamine interaction: Relevance to Parkinson's disease. Prog. Neuro-Psychopharmacol. and Biol. Psychiat., 17, 139-150.

Benson, B. (1999). Pineal Gland Neuropeptides. In R.R. Watson (ed.), Melatonin in the Promotion of Health (pp. 137-149). Boca Raton, FL: CRC Press, Inc.

Berardesca, E., de Rigal, Leveque, J.L. and Maibach, H.I. (1991). *In vivo* biophysical characterization of skin physiological differences in races. Dermatologica, 182(2), 89-93.

Binkley, S., Riebman, J. and Reilly, K. (1977). Timekeeping by the pineal gland. Science, 197, 1181-1183.

Binkley, S. (1988). The Pineal: Endocrine and Nonendocrine Function. New Jersey: Prentice Hall.

Blois, M.S. (1969). In F. Urbach (ed.), The Biological Effects of Ultraviolet Radiation. New York: Pergamon.

Blois, M.S. (1971). In T. Kawamura, T.B. Fitzparick, M. Seiji (Eds.), Biology of Normal and Abnormal Melanocytes. Baltimore: University Press.

Bogerts, B. (1981). A brainstem atlas of catecholaminergic neurons in man, using melanin as a natural marker. Journal of Comparative Neurology, 197, 63-80.

Boissy, R.E., Zhao, H., Oetting, W.S., Austin, L.M., Wildenberg, S.C., Boissy, Y.L., Zhao, Y., Sturm, R.A., Hearing, V.J., King, R.A. and Norlund, J.J. (1996). Mutation and lack of expression of tyrosinase-related protein-1 (TRP-1) in melanocytes from an invidual with brown oculocutaneous albinism: A new subtype of albinism classified as "OCA3." American Journal of Human Genetics, 58, 1145-1156.

Buffey, J.A., Hill, S.E., Bleehen, S.S., Thody, A.J. and MacNeil, S. (1991). Evidence for a calcium/calmodulin involvement in density-dependent melanogenesis in murine B16 melanoma cells. Pigment Cell Research, 4, 112-119.

Bustamante, J., Bredeston, L., Malanga, G. and Mordoh, J. (1993). Role of melaniin as a scavenger of active oxygen species. Pigment Cell Research, 6, 348-353.

Bynum, E.B. (1999). African Unconscious: Roots of Ancient Mysticism and Modern Psychology.
New York: Teachers College Press.

Caroff, S.N. (1980). The neuroleptic malignant syndrome. Journal of Clinical Psychiatry, 41, 79-83.

Carstam, R., Brinck, C., Hindemith-Augustsson, A., Rorsman, H. And Rosengren, V. (1991). The neuromelanin of the substantia nigra. Biochim. Biophys. Acta., 1097, 152-160.

Carter, N.L. (1980). Eye color and susceptibility to noise-induced permanent threshold shift. Audiology, 19, 86-93.

Carter, N.L., Keen, K., Waugh, R.L., Murray, N. and Bulteau, V.G. (1981). The relationship of eye color and noise-induced permanent threshold shift. Audiology, 20, 336-346.

Chandler, W.B. (1999). Ancient Future: The Teachings and Prophetic Wisdom of the Seven Hermetic Laws of Ancient Egypt. Baltimore, MD: Black Classic Press.

Chhajlani, V. and Wikberg, J.E.S. (1992). Molecular cloning and expression of the human melanocyte stimulating hormone receptor cDNA. FEBS Letter, 309, 417-420.

Cohen, G. (1987). Oxygen radicals and Parkinson's disease. In Upjohn Symposium/Oxygen Radicals.

Commoner, B., Townsend, J. and Pake G.E. (1954). Free radicals in biological materials. Nature, 174, 689-691.

Conlee, J.W., Abdul-Baqi, K.J., McCandles, G.A., and Creel, D.J. (1986). Differential susceptibility to noise-induced permanent threshold shift between albino and pigmented guinea pigs. Hearing Research, 23, 81-91.

Conlee, J.W., Abdul-Baqi, K.J., McCandles, G.A., and Creel, D.J. (1988). Effects of aging on normal hearing loss and noise-induced threshold shift in albino and pigmented guinea pigs. Acta Otolaryngol., 106, 64-70.

Conlee, J.W., Gerity, L.C., Westenberg, I.S. and Creel, D.J. (1994). Pigment-dependent differences in the stria vascularis of albino and pigmented guinea pigs and rats. Hearing Research, 72, 108-124.

Conlee, J.W., Benett, M.L. and Creel, D.J. (1995). Differential effects of gentamicin on the distribution of cochlear function in albino and pigmented guinea pigs. Acta Otolaryngol., 115, 367-374.

Constantinescu, C.S. (1995). Melanin, melatonin, melanocyte-stimulating hormone, and the susceptibility to autoimmune demyelination: a rationale for light therapy in multple sclerosis. Medical Hypothesis, 45(5), 455-458.

Cooper, R.J., Bloom, F.E. and Roth, R.H. (1991). The Biochemical Basis of Neuropharmacology. Oxford, England: Oxford University Press.

Cowley, G. (1995 August 7). Can melatonin stop the clock? Newsweek, pp. 46-49.

Cross, C.E., et al. (1987). Oxygen radicals and human disease. Annals in Internal Medicine, 107, 526-545.

Danielczyk, W. et al. (1988). Platelet MAO B activity and the psychopathology of Parkinson's disease, senile dementia and multi-infarct dementia. Acta Psychiatr. Scand., 78, 730-736.

Descartes, R. (1649). Les Passions de l'ame. In J.Reeves (Ed.). Body and Mind in Western Thought (pp. 293-294). New York: Penguin Books, 1950.

Ebadi, M. and Govitrapong, P. (1986). Orphan transmitters and their receptors. In R.J. Reiter, Pineal Research Reviews, Vol. 4. New York: Alan R. Liss.

Ebadi, M., Hexum, T.D., Pfeiffer, R.F. and Govitrapong, P. (1989). Pineal and retinal peptides and their receptors. In R.J. Reiter, Pineal Research Reviews, Vol. 4. New York: Alan R. Liss.

Ekmehag, B., Persson, B., Rorsman, P. and Rorsman, H. (1994). Demonstration of voltage-dependent and TTX-sensitive Na+-channels in human melanocytes. Pigment Cell Research, 7, 333-338.

Enochs, W.S., Sarna, T., Zecca, L., Riley, P.A. and Swartz, H.M. (1994). The role of neuromelanin, binding of metal ions, and oxidative cytotoxicity in the pathogenesis of Parkinson's disease: a hypothesis. Journal of Neural Transmission: Parkinson's Disease Dementia Section, 7(2), 83-100.

Faraldi, F., Reyes, M.G., Alfieri, E. and Levi, A.C. (1994). The aging substantia nigra: quantitative histologic study. Panminerva Med, 73(2), 103-108.

Farooqui, J.Z., Medrano, E.E., Abdel-Malek, Z. and Norlund, J. (1993). The expression of proopiomelanocortin and various POMC-derived peptides in mouse and human skin. Annals in the New York Academy of Sciences, 680, 508-510.

Fitzpatrick, T.B. and Breathnach, A.S. (1963). Das epidermale melanin-einheit system. Derm. Wochenschr, 147, 481-489.

Foley, J.M. and Baxter,D. (1958). On the nature of pigment granules in the cells of the locus coeruleus and substantia nigra. Journal of Neuropathology and Experimental Neurology, 17, 586-598.

Freedman, D. (1998). The Mysterious Middle of the Milky Way. Discover (November), pp. 66-75.

Fuller, B.B. (1987). Inhibition of tyrosinase activity and protein synthesis in melanoma cells by calcium ionophore A23187. Pigment Cell Research, 1, 176-180.

Gertz, H.J. and Schmidt, L.G. (1991). Low melanin content of substantia nigra in a case of neuroleptic malignant syndrome. Pharmacopsychiat., 24, 93-95.

Golbe, L.I., Cody, R.A. and Duvoisin, R.C. (1986). Smoking and Parkinson's disease. Search for a dose-response relationship. Archives in Neurology, 43, 774-778.

Golbe, L.I. et al. (1990). A large kindred with autosomal dominant Parkinson's disease. Archives in Neurology, 27, 276-282.

Graham, D.G. (1978). Oxidative pathways for catecholamines in the genesis of neuromelanin and cytotoxic quinones. Molecular Pharmacology, 14, 633-643.

Grant, W.C. (1961). Special aspects of the metamorphic process: second metamorphis. American Zoology, 1, 163-171.

Greenwell, B. (1990). Energies of Transformation: A Guide to the Kundalini Process. Shakti River Press.

Hadley, M.E. et al. (1996). Melanocortin receptors: Identification and characterization of melanotropic peptide agonists and antagonists. Pigment Cell Research, 9, 213-234.

Hill, S.E., Buffey, J., Thody, A.J., Oliver, I., Bleehen, S.S. and MacNeil, S. (1989). Investigation of the regulation of pigmentation in á-melanocyte-stimulating hormone responsive and unresponsive cultured B16 melanoma cells. Pigment Cell Research, 2, 161-166.

Hille, B. (1992). Ionic channels of excitable membranes (2nd Ed.). Sunderland, MA: Sinauer Associates, Inc.

Hoffman, M. (1995). Some old genes just don't quit. American Scientist, 83, 235-236.

Holick, M.F. (1985). The photobiology of vitamin D and its consequences for humans. In R.J. Wurtman, M.J. Baum and J.T. Potts (Eds.). The medical and biological effects of light, Annals of The New York Academy of Sciences, Volume 453, (pp. 1-13).

Hood, J., Poole, J.P. and Freeman, L. (1976). The influence of eye color upon temporary threshold shift. Audiology, 15, 238-243.

Hruby, V.J. et al. (1996). Cyclic lactam alpha-melanotropin analogues of Ac-Nle4-c[Asp4,D-phe7,Lys10] alpha-MSH(4-10)-NH2 with bulky aromatic amino acids at position 7 show high antagonist potency and selectivity at melanocortin receptors. Journal of Medicinal Chemistry, 38, 3454-3461.

Huda, A. et al. (1984). Endogenous opioid peptides: Biology and functions. Annual Reviews in Neuroscience, 7, 223-255.

Humfrey, C.D.N. et al. (1990). Monoamine oxidase substrates in Parkinson's disease. Biochemical Pharmacology, 40, 2562-2564.

Hunt, G., Donatien, P.D., Lunec, J., Todd, C., Kyne, S. and Thody, A.J. (1994). Cultured human melanocytes respond to MSH peptides and ACTH. Pigment Cell Research, 7, 217-221.

Inzelberg, R., Flash, T. Schechtman, E. and Korczyn, A.D. (1995). Kinematic properties of upper limb trajectories in idiopathic torsion dystonia. Journal of Neurology, Neurosurgery and Psychiatry, 58, 312-319.

Ito, S. (1993). Biochemistry and physiology of melanin. In N. Levine (Ed.). Pigmentation and Pigmentary Disorders (pp. 33-59). Boca Raton, FL: CRC Press.

Iyengar, B. and Misra, R.S. (1988). The neural differentiation of melanocytes in vitiliginous skin. Acta Anatomica, 133, 62-65.

Iyengar, B. (1995). Corticotropin expression by human melanocytes in the skin. Pigment Cell Research, 8, 142-146.

James, G.G.M. (1954). Stolen Legacy. San Francisco, CA: Julian Richardson Associates.

Jaroff, L. (1994, April 4). Teaching reverse racism. TIME, pp. 74-75.

Jet Magazine (1995 June 26). Why Blacks age better than Whites. pp. 24-26.

Jenner, P. (1992). What process causes nigral cell death in Parkinson's disease. Neurologic Clinics, 10(2), 387-403.

Jiang, J., Sharma, S.D., Hruby, V.J., Bentley, D.L., Fink, J.L. and Hadley, M.E. (1996). Human epidermal melanocyte and keratinocyte melanocortin receptors: Visualization by melanotropic peptide conjugated microshperes (Latex Beads). Pigment Cell Research, 9, 240-247.

Kahn, M., Pepose, J.S., Green, W.R., Miller, J. and Foos, R.Y. (1993). Immunocytologic findings in a case of Vogt-Koyanagi-Harada syndrome. Opthalmology, 100, 1191-1198.

Kambon, K.K. (1998). African/Black Psychology in the American Context: An African-Centered Approach. Tallahassee, FL: Nubian Nation Publications.

Kaiya, H. (1980). Neuromelanin, neuroleptics and schizophrenia. Neuropsychobiology, 6, 241-248.

Kimura, H., Ohashi, N., Aso, S. and Watanabe, Y. (1996). Clinical study of the role of melanocytes in the inner ear of patients with Harada's disease. ORL, 58, 233-237.

King, R. (1990). African Origin of Biological Psychiatry. Tennessee: Seymour-Smith Inc.

King, R. (1994). Melanin: A Key to Freedom. Hampton, VA: U.B. & U.S. Communications Systems, Inc.

King, R., Locke, G.E., King, L.M., Miles, R. and Thompson, N. (1994). The Pineal Gland, Melanin, and Calcium: Pineal Gland Calcification in African-Americans - A Review of 1,622 Cases. Hampton, VA: U.B. & U.S. Communications Systems, Inc.

Kittles, R. (1995). Nature, origin, and variation of human pigmentation. Journal of Black Studies, 26(1), 36-61.

Kippenberger, S., Bernd, A., Bereiter-Hahn, J., Ramirez-Bosca, A., Kaufman, R. and Holzmann, H. (1996). Transcription of melanogenesis enzymes in melanocytes: Dependence upon culture conditions and co-cultivation with keratinocytes. Pigment Cell Research, 9, 179-184.

Lacy, M.E. (1984). Phonon-electron coupling as a possible transducing mechanism in bioelectronic processes involving neuromelanin. Journal of Theoretical Biology, 111, 201-204.

Langston, J.W., Ballard, P. and Tetrud, J.W. (1983). Chronic parkinsonism in humans due to a product of meperidine-analogue synthesis. Science, 219, 979-980.

Larsson, B. and Tjalve, H. (1979). Studies on the mechanisms of drug-binding to melanin. Biochemical Pharmacology, 28, 1181-1187.

Larsson, B.S. (1993). Interaction between chemicals and melanin. Pigment Cell Research, 6, 127-133.

Le Douarin, N.M. and Kalcheim, C. (1999). The Neural Crest (2nd Ed). New York: Cambridge University Press.

Lerner, A.B., Case, J.D., Takahashi, Y, Lee, T.H. and Mori, W. (1958). Isolation of melatonin, the pineal gland factor that lightens melanocytes. Journal of American Chemical Society, 80, 2587.

Lindquist, N.G., Larsson, B.S. and Lyden-Sokolowski, A. (1987). Neuromelanin and its possible protective and destructive properties. Pigment Cell Research, 1, 133-136.

Maeda, K., Naganuma, M., Fukuda, M., Matsunaga, J. and Tomita, Y. (1996). Effect of pituitary and ovarian hormones on human melanocytes *in vitro*. Pigment Cell Research, 9, 204-212.

Mann, D.M.A. and Yates, P.O. (1974). Lipoprotein pigments- their relationship to aging in th human nervous system. II. The melanin content of pigmented nerve cells. Brain, 97, 489-498.

Marsden, C.D. (1983). Neuromelanin and parkinson's disease. Journal of Neural Transmission, 19, 121-141.

McGinness, J. (1972). Mobility gaps: A mechanism for band gaps in melanins. Science, 177, 896.

McGinness, J. and Proctor, P. (1973). The importance of the fact that melanin is black Journal of Theoretical Biology, 39, 677-688.

McGinness, J., Corry, P. and Proctor, P. (1974). Amorphous semiconductor switching in melanins. Science, 183, 853-855.

Moore, T.O. (1995). The Science of Melanin: Dispelling the Myths. Silver Spring, MD: Beckham House Publishers.

Moore, T.O. (1996). Melatonin Mania. Psych Disourse, 27(2), 4-10.

Moore, T.O. (1997). Historical challenges to maintaining health in African American males. Challenge: A Journal of Research on African American Men, 8 (1), 45-57.

Mountjoy, K.G., Robbins, L.S., Mortrud, M.T. and Cone, R.D. (1992). The cloning of a family of genes that encode the melanocortin receptors. Science, 257, 1248-1251.

Nakamura, S. et al. (1996). Melanin-laden macrophages in cerebrospinal fluid in Vogt-Koyanagi-Harada syndrome. Archives in Opthalmology, 114, 1184-1188.

Nash, J.M. (1997). Addicted: Why do some people get hooked? Mounting evidence points to a powerful brain chemical called dopamine. Time, 149(18), May 5, pp. 1-7.

Newsweek (2000 September 18). Redefining race in America. pp. 38-65.

Newsweek (2000 November 26). Pigment in a Tube. pp. 86.

Nilius, B., Bohm, T. and Wohlrab, W. (1990). Properties of a potassium-selective ion channel in human melanoma cells. Pflugers Arch., 417, 269-277.

Nilius, B. and Wohlrab, W. (1992). Potassium channels and regulation of proliferation of human melanoma cells. Journal of Physiology, 445, 537-548.

Okada, T. et al. (1996). Vitiligo in Vogt-Koyanagi-Harada disease: immunohistological analysis of inflammatory site. Graefes Arch. Clin. Exp. Opthalmol., 234, 359-363.

Pawelek, J.M. et al. (1992). Molecular cascades in UV-induced melanogenesis: A central role for melanotropins? Pigment Cell Research, 5, 348-356.

Percival, H.W. (1974). Thinking and Destiny: Being the Science of Man. Dallas, TX: The World Foundation, Inc.

Pfeiffer, C.C. and Mailloux, R.J. (1988). Hypertension: heavy metals, useful cations and melanin as a possible repository. Medical Hypothesis, 26(2), 125-130.

Polymeropoulos, M.H. et al. (1996). Mapping of a gene for Parkinson's disease to chromosome 4q21-q23. Science, 274, 1197-1199.

Pookrum, J. (1993). Vitamins and Minerals from A to Z. Brooklyn, NY: A&BBooks Publishers.

Price, S.L. (1997a). What ever happened to the White athlete? Sports Illustrated, December 8, pp. 31-51.

Price, S.L. (1997b). Is it in the genes? Sports Illustrated, December 8, pp. 53-54.

Prota, G. (1992). Melanins and Melanogenesis. San Diego, CA: Academic Press.

Rada, L.G., Venturelli, F. and Roscetti, G. (1986). Hydrolysis and protection from hydrolysis of circulating enkephalins. Comparative Biochemistry and Physiology, 85C, 449-454.

Rao, N.A., Moorthy, R.S. and Inomata, H. (1995). Vogt-Koyanagi-Harada syndrome. Int. Opthalmol.Clin., 35, 69-86.

Rodgers, A.D. and Curzon, G. (1975). Melanin formation by human brain in vitro. Journal of Neurochemistry, 24 1123-1129.

Rosei, M.A., Blarzino, C., Foppoli, C., Mosca, L. and Coccia, R. (1994). Lipoxygenase-catalyzed oxidation of catecholamines. Biochem. Biophys. Res. Commun., 200, 344-350.

Rosei, M.A., Mosca, L., Foppoli, C., Coccia, R. and De Marco, C. (1995). Alternative enzymes in melanin synthesis. Melanoma Research, 5, 24.

Rosei, M.A. (1996). Melanins from opioid peptides. Pigment Cell Research, 9, 273-280.

Rosenthal, N.E., Sack, D., Gillin, J.C., Lewy, A.J., Goodwin, F.K., Davenport, Y., Mueller, P.S., Newsome, D.A. and Wehr, T. (1984). Seasonal affective disorder: A Description of the syndrome and preliminary findings with light therapy. Archives in General Psychiatry, 41, 72-80.

Rubin, V. (1998, March). Dark matter in the universe. Scientific American, 1-7.

Shalev, A. and Munitz, H. (1986). The neuroleptic malignant syndrome: Agent and host interaction. Acta Psychiatr. Scand., 73, 337-347.

Shima, T. et al. (1997). Binding of iron to neuromelanin of human substantia nigra and synthetic melanin: an electron paramagnetic resonance spectroscopy study. Free Radical Biological Medicine, 73(1), 110.

Sian, J., Youdim, M.B.H., Riederer, P. and Gerlach, M. (1999). Neurotransmitters and disorders of the basal ganglia. In G.J. Siegel et al. (Eds), Basic Neurochemistry: Molecular, Cellular and Medical Aspects (pp. 917-947). New York: Lippincott, Williams and Wilkins.

Slominski, A., Costantino, R., Wortsman, J., Paus, R. and Ling, N. (1992). Melanotropic activity of gamma MSH peptides in melanoma cells. Life Science, 50, 1103-1108.

Smythies, J.R. (1996). On the functional role of neuromelanin. Proc. R. Soc. Lond. B. Biol. Sci., 263(1369), 487-489.

Smythies, J.R. (1997). Oxidative reactions and schizophrenia: a review-discussion. Schizophrenia Research, 24(3), 357-364.

Stark, P., Fuller, R.W. and Wong, D.T. (1985). The pharmacologic profile of fluoxetine. Journal of Clinical Psychiatry, 46(3), 7-13.

Stumpf, W.E. (1988). The endocrinology of sunlight and darkness: complimentary roles of vitamin D and pineal hormones. Naturwissenschaften, 75, 247-251.

Stumpf, W.E. and Privette, T.H. (1989). Light, vitamin D and psychiatry: role of 1,25 dihydroxyvitamin D3 (soltriol) in etiology and therapy of seasonal affective disorder and other mental processes. Psychopharmacology, 97, 285-294.

Sugita, S. et al. (1996). Melanocyte lysis by cytotoxic T lymphocytes recognizing the MART-1 melanoma antigen in HLA-A2 patients with Vogt-Koyanagi-Harada disease. Intern. Immunol., 8, 799-803.

Tachibana, M. (1999). Sound needs sound melanocytes to be heard. Pigment Cell Research, 12, 344-354.

Tanner, C.M., Cohen, J.C., Summerville, B.C. and Goetz, C.G. (1988). Vitamin use and Parkinson's disease. Annals in Neurology, 233, 182.

Tanner, C.M. (1992). Epidemiology of Parkinson's disease. Neurologics, 10(2), 317-329.

Tobin, D., Quinn. A.G., Ito, S. and Thody, A.J. (1994). The presence of tyrosinase and related proteins in human epidermis and their relationship to melanin type. Pigment Cell Research, 7, 204-209.

Tomita, Y., Fukushima, M. and Tagami, H. (1986). Stimulation of melanogenesis by cholecalciferol in cultured human melanocytes: a possible mechanism underlying pigmentation after ultraviolet irradiation. Tohoku Journal of Experimental Medicine, 149, 451-452.

Tota, G. and Bocci, G. (1967). Importance of the color of the iris in the evaluation of resistance of hearing to fatigue. Reviews in Otoneuroophtalmology, 43, 183-192.

Trefil, J. (1993). Dark matter. Smithsonian, 24(3), 27-35.

Vivien-Roels, B., Masson-Pevet. M., Canguilhem, B., Bonn, D., and Pevet, P. (1993). Effect of photoperiod on the daily rhythm of pineal and/or circulating melatonin and 5-methoxytryptophol (ML) concentrations in the European hamster *Cricetus cricetus*. In Y, Touitou, J. Arendt amd P. Pevet (Eds.). Melatonin and the Pineal Gland - From Basic Science to Clinical Application. Amsterdam: Elsevier.

Vriend, J. (1983). Evidence for pineal gland modulation of the neuroendocrine-thyroid axis. Neuroendocrinology, 36, 68-78.

Watson, R.R. (1999). Melatonin in the Promotion of Health. Boca Raton, FL: CRC Press, Inc.

Welsing, F.C. (1991). The Isis Papers: The Keys to the Colors. Chicago: Third World Press.

Willis, C. (1994). The skin we're in. Discover, November, 76-81.

Wintzen, M. and Gilchrest, B.A. (1996). Proopiomelanocortin, its derived peptides, and the skin. Journal of Investigative Dermatology, 106, 3-10.

Wurtman, R.J. and Axelrod, J. (1965). The Pineal gland. Scientific American, 213, 50-60.

Wurtman, R.J., Axelrod, J. and Kelly, D.E. (1968). The Pineal. New York: Academic Press.

Yamane, H. et al. (1995). Appearance of free radicals in the guinea pig inner ear after noise-induced acoustic trauma. Eur. Arch. Otolaryngol., 252, 504-508.

Yoon, C.K. (1996). New light on seasonal disorder (SAD) therapy. Journal of NIH Research, 8, 29-31.

Youdim, M.B., Ben-Shachar, D. and Riederer. (1994). The enigma of neuromelanin in Parkinson's disease substantia nigra. Journal of Neural Transmission, Suppl, 73(2), 113-122.

Young, V.W. and Perry, T.L. (1986). Monoamine oxidase B, smoking and Parkinson's disease. Journal of Neurological Science, 72, 265-272.

Zagon, I.S., Wu, Y. And McLaughlin, P.J. (1996). The opioid growth factor met-enkephalin and zeta opioid receptor are present in human and mouse skin tonically act to inhibit DNA synthesis in the epidermis. Journal of Investigative Dermatology, 106, 490-497.

Zamir, N., Palkovits, M., Weber, E., Mezey, E. and Brownstein, M.J. (1984). A dynorphinergic pathway of Leu-enkephalin production in rat substantia nigra. Nature, 307, 643-645.

Zecca, L. et al. (1994). Iron and other metals in neuromelanin, substantia nigra, and putamen of human brain. Journal of Neurochemistry, 73(2), 1097-1101.

Zecca, L. et al. (1996). Interaction of neuromelanin and iron in substantia nigra and other areas of human brain. Neuroscience, 73(2), 407-415.

DARK SECRETS

INTRODUCTION

Drugs are external agents that can significantly alter human behavior. In *Dark Secrets*, we will address drug addiction from a quite different perspective. We will discuss drug addiction and melanin research in the context of genetic and ethnic variations. Drug addiction is a severe problem that can incapacitate an individual from functioning in society. The drugs which specifically affect the neurotransmitter dopamine are the pharmacological agents we will highlight. All humans have similar internal mechanisms that can cause addiction. No matter what cultural group or ethnic background one may come from, addiction does not discriminate. We would be naive to believe, however, that there are no physical anomalies related to why some people may experience addiction differently. Although there are other biological factors to consider (Strickland and Gray, 2000), it is the differences related to melanin that stimulates the impetus for writing this book.

Scientists have used a sociological concept (i.e., race) to define differences in the past, but "race" is useless when you understand the origins of humanity. If there is a race, then it is the human race. Many "endarkened" scholars are no longer blinded by the white light of Eurocentrism, and now have a scientific understanding that Africa is the origin of *Homo sapien sapiens*. Genetically speaking, all human beings on the planet are biological derivatives from the darkly pigmented inhabitants from Africa.

It is this ancient African source of melanin that has created the current biopsychosocial politics of melanin research. Since people of African descent have been historically disrespected by nonpigmented scientists, it becomes a political statement to denigrate rather than elevate anything related to blackness. For example, western education has led us to believe that dark-skinned African people contributed nothing of significance to humanity. A Eurocentric perspective of history and science would find little value in concepts, issues and topics related to blackness. Until alternative viewpoints are provided, melanin research may be difficult to interpret.

In Part Two (*Dark Secrets*), we will expose the societal problems that cause people to be seduced by drugs. Everyone has the potential to become addicted to drugs, but the assault on the African American community has been relentless. The psychosocial issues associated with drug addiction are explicitly presented in Chapter 6- The Pacification Process and Addiction. The thoughts and ideas of the late Dr. Amos Wilson are resurrected, along with analyses from the work of Dr. Frances Cress Welsing. In my opinion, Amos Wilson has given the most clear critique on how Western society has created addictive personalities in the African American community. We will extend his ideas and present a common view that addiction is really a disease in Chapter 7 - Thinking of Addiction as a Disease. As we course through literature suggesting that addiction is a disease, Chapter 8- Melanin and Drug Binding will highlight the physical effects of drug addiction on melinated systems. Chapter 9 - An Internal Imbalance will highlight the analogy that addiction is like throwing away the lock and key. There is much scientific evidence to suggest that dopamine is the rewarding molecule that stimulates pleasure. Throwing away the lock and key suggests that drugs can permanently alter dopamine (the key) levels and dopamine receptors (lock), and subsequently, lock you into a perpetual state of addiction. In conclusion, Chapter 10 - Dark Secrets Revealed, we will uncover the fact that biologically, there are ethnic differences in the response to certain drugs. In addition, we will consider a drug abuse prevention model that can promote a positive perspective on health.

To respect your self and your body, you must first know your self and your body. Addiction results when people disrespect themselves or if they have poor relationships with others. To fully prevent drug addiction, the echoes of our African ancestors still reverberate - KNOW THYSELF. Prepare yourself for another "endarkening" experience.

T. Owens Moore
January 8, 2001

Chapter 6

The Pacification Process and Addiction

Addiction can occur in many forms. You can be addicted to material items, other people, hobbies and pharmacological agents (e.g., drugs). In *Dark Secrets*, the focus is solely on drug addiction and how addictive-type personalities can be created. A sociopolitical analysis will be provided to explore how the mind can be manipulated and how behavior can be pacified and controlled with drugs. In reference to "dark matter," we are referring to people of African descent and how their behavior can be manipulated on a mass scale.

The physical, mental and spiritual bondage that was experienced by African people during American slavery has greatly attributed to the poor state of affairs in the African American community. Invaders to the continent of Africa and ruthless foreigners from the Western world have exploited African people for many centuries. It is a sad human predicament, but it is the color of skin that has caused so much sociopolitical grief. Nonpigmented individuals have used skin color as a curse to hold down people of African descent. Do not believe that African people were subjugated solely for their pigmented skin, however. The truth of the matter is that they were physically far superior than other ethnic/cultural groups who were unable to endure the harsh realities of slavery (Semmes, 1996). The capitalism of slavery needed a strong work force, not a colorfully pigmented group of slaves. What is totally perverse today is that it is the pigment of a person's skin that has hindered the positive development of human social relations. The falsified Hamitic curse still exists.

Dark-skinned people of African descent have a long history of being subjugated by people with less pigment in their skin. There are a plethora of reasons for the world-wide degradation of dark-skinned Africans and their culture, but the mere color of their skin is the most visible factor (see Welsing, 1991). Frances Cress Welsing, a prominent African American psychiatrist, has presented a dynamic analysis of how nonpigmented or white people have managed to control the world through a white supremacists ideology. Dr. Welsing's Cress Theory of Color Confrontation and Racism can be used as an example to explain the relationship between skin color and social subjugation.

The Cress Theory of Color Confrontation and Racism states that:

> "...the color-deficient Europeans responded psychologically, with a profound sense of numerical inadequacy and color inferiority, in their confrontations with the majority of the world's people - all of whom possessed varying degrees of color-producing capacity. This psychological response, whether conscious or unconscious, revealed an inadequacy based on the most obvious and fundamental part of their being, their external appearance. As might be anticipated in terms of modern psychological theories, whites defensively developed an uncontrollable sense of hostility and aggression" p. 4.

According to Welsing, "the perplexing psychological reaction of whites has been directed towards all peoples with the capacity to produce melanin." In the past twenty years, reflect on the locations where the U.S. military excursions have occurred (Grenada, Panama, Somalia, Haiti and Iraq). Other than military excursions, manipulating the minds of the people is another effective way to control and subjugate people.

Since the "Black Revolution" of the 1960s, the U.S. government has done very little to curtail drug trafficking and the use and abuse of drugs in the U.S., especially the African American community (Lusane, 1991). It is not suggested that African Americans are the only group of people to experience drug use and abuse, but the controlling effect of drugs is highlighted by the way the government used drugs to quiet the Black Revolution. Since the physical shackles of slavery were no longer binding African people to the system, drugs were later used as an effective way to pacify any rebellious behavior. A certain type of personality needed to be created and the research from behavioral scientists such as Dr. Burris F. Skinner were indirectly used by the controlling powers to quiet the masses. As analyzed by the late Dr. Bobby Wright, Skinner wrote *Beyond Freedom and Dignity* in 1971 to demonstrate how behavior could be controlled without you being aware. Skinner's book was written after the 1960s, but a careful reading of this document can suggest how the government could pass civil rights legislation and still effectively control the people who were requesting their rights. This social construct called "Negro" and the mentality it generated has come back to haunt us forever because it set the stage for a passive personality that could be easily persuaded to look outside of self for solutions.

Integration has nearly destroyed the moral code that pervaded many African American communities in the past. To be specific, integration was actually assimilation because White Americans did not choose to move into black communities. Even in 2001, when Blacks move into predominantly white neighborhoods, White Americans appear to have an innate response that causes them to slowly uproot and move further away. It is their choice to do so, but it magnifies the fact that integration is a farce. Assimilation is more accurate to explain how African Americans are ass emulating (i.e., assimilate) someone else who has utter disdain for them. A respectable socioeconomic status of the Black neighbors may make no difference because the dreaded curse of pigmented skin can make insecure nonpigmented people feel xenophobic. Our discussion is not on the collective psyche of white behavior because this has been detailed elsewhere (Welsing, 1991; Forbes, 1992; Ani, 1994; Bradley, 1991). Our focus is on the personalities created by ass emulation.

In Western society, materialism is the defining factor which determines ones existence. Being able to control and dominate your environment is paramount to a Western way of viewing the world. According to Dr. Amos Wilson (1990), African American desires, tastes, and needs are so evoked and organized by White American manufactured products, marketing strategies and social status concepts that their attempted and accomplished satisfaction maintains the very system which oppresses them. This analysis profoundly influences addictive behavior because African Americans consume deadly substances directly marketed to them (e.g., malt liquor and crack cocaine) by White America. Wilson expounds in the following manner:

> "Through its manipulation of production and prices it seeks to manipulate the social conditions and the organization (as well as disorganization) of the behavior, perception and consciousness of those who seek to acquire what it produces. Its production methods and organization sustain the status quo and the system of values and social relations, which support its hegemony " p.137.

Without the addicts desire, the organizational structure of the drug culture and the White organizational structure would not exist. Therefore, an addictive personality must be maintained by the White organizational structure to keep African Americans and any other threatening group in a perpetual state of control. If you are bold, strong, viable and resilient, then you are a threat to insecure people.

In today's society, it is quite masterful how previously bold Black male behavior has been manipulated and pacified. In the pacification process, multiple aberrant forms of behavior may result. Although Wilson (1990) provided a brilliant analysis of the psychodynamics of black self-annihilation in service of white domination, Welsing (1991) has also provided incite to the cycle of violence centered around the drug culture:

> "The chain of events begins with the denial of full scale employment and advancement to Black males so that they cannot adequately support themselves, their wives and their children. In turn, large numbers of Black male children grow up without their father's guidance. This leads to frustra tion, depression and failure in school. Once this atmosphere is established, drugs are placed *deliberately* in the Black com munity. The drugs are then used to "street treat" Black male frustration and depression. The high prices for which drugs

are sold provide the Black male population with the *illusion* that finally they are beginning to make some money and to share in the "American Dream." Guns are then placed at the disposal of the same Black male persons, supposedly to aid them in enforcing payment for drug sales. More important, the strategy is for Black males to kill and destroy one another and then carry the blame. (It must be realized that no Black males manufacture the chemicals for drug use, nor do any Black males manufacture guns.)" p. iv.

Besides the many social implications, long-term use of drugs of abuse can lead to a physical condition called addiction. The power of drug addiction is so overwhelming that it can be influenced by media advertisements (external source) or from a physical change in a person's biological structure (internal source). In this chapter, we are interested in the manufactured external forces that affect the thinking of African people. Accordingly, an addict will value and devalue persons relative to his/her addictions, and what the addict values is instigated by both external and internal forces.

There is a real psychology to addiction that totally destroys the capacity for self-control, and loss of self-control can begin innocently with the consumption of alcohol. In terms of African American youth, it is criminal the way some youth are targeted for alcohol consumption. Powell (1995), for example, reviewed the scandalous nature of marketing malt liquor to African American youth. Miseducated African American youth are seduced into consuming 40 ounces of malt liquor versus other alcoholic drinks because the advertisements for malt liquor thrive on sex and power for marketing (Powell, 1995)

Since human behavior is far more oriented and regulated by anticipations, temptations, enticements and incentives, than by internal drives, needs or deprivations, it is simple to see how African Americans or any other oppressed group of people can be controlled in this society. By not manufacturing or controlling anything life-saving or life-giving (Mahabuti, 1978) post-integration, African

Americans have ass emulated and set themselves up to be controlled by external forces. Human behavior is more "pulled" than "pushed," i.e., impelled by external forces and their internal representations than the other way around (Wilson, 1990). Therefore, it is easy to see how images of sex and power could be used to successfully distribute a deadly ethnic specific product (e.g., malt liquor) to African Americans.

Excessive consumption of alcohol can have a detrimental effect on the brain, but the physiological effects of 40 ounces of malt liquor on the brain of a young person can be considerably harmful (Moore, 1997). Malt liquor consumption may lead to numerous social maladjustments and increase the desire to consume illegal drugs. In general, the brain acts to inhibit behavior and large amounts of alcohol tend to have a depressant effect on the brain. The result is disinhibition. This means that inhibitions a person normally experiences will weaken or disappear when they consume liquid crack (i.e., malt liquor). Although speculative, it is possible that malt liquor can make men more sexually aggressive and women more accommodating.

American society alienates African Americans from themselves and their culture, and this lack of self-knowledge feeds addictive behavior. If you truly knew who you were, there is no way one could engage in self-destructive behavior. In addition to specific groups of miseducated African Americans, any poor or oppressed cultural group in America is a prime target for creating addictive-type personalities. Wilson (1990) states:

> "The racial/class hierarchy in America is maintained through the White American maintenance of large discrepancies between the objects of desire they produce and the means by which they are obtained. Gross imbalances between means and ends, between expectations and the possibilities of their fulfillment, are endemic to American society. It does little, if anything, to prepare its citizens to fulfill the expectations it socializes into them, or to provide them with wholesome and affordable means of self-fulfillment" p. 139.

In sum, there is no mystery why addiction is so pervasive in society. Whether you are rich or from the middle-class or underclass, the addictive properties of drugs do not discriminate across socioeconomic status. For the purpose of our discussion on the pacification process and addiction, it is the miseducated underclass that may be most affected by the negative effects of the drug culture. Some poor people with no vision or purpose in life are prone to waddle their worries into an external substance rather than gain self-control and find solutions to their problems. The biopsychosocial politics arise when poor people are ingesting unhealthy substances and simultaneously supporting an exploitative economy. The irrational economy of White America, based as it is on irrational consumption, requires a high level of impulsivity and economic stupidity in its population (Wilson, 1990). Poor people who have no money will find a way to support a drug habit and willfully neglect to handle their personal matters (e.g., family, household, bills). The impact of addiction is devastating and it is now understood that it has a biological source. As we will discuss in the next chapter, addiction is a brain disease.

Chapter 7

Thinking of Addiction as a Disease

The brain is a malleable organ and brain function is dependent on internal as well as external factors. By thinking of drug addiction as a disease, we are focusing on the internal mechanisms that are transformed or altered. These internal changes can cause permanent alterations in the brain and create an imbalanced mental state. Addiction is the result of the brain attempting to regain the altered state created by the drug. Dis-ease terminology is used because the brain is not at ease, but in an abnormal state.

As I have emphasized before (Moore, 1995), our bodies are a microcosm of the macrocosm, and we are intimately connected to nature in many ways. The human body has a very similar chemical composition to the planet we live on and numerous plants found in nature have chemical substances which are also found in our body. Therefore, our internal anatomy can be influenced by substances found in the external environment. Many of the hallucinogenic substances found in plants and mushrooms, for example, have chemical properties that mimic the effects of natural brain chemicals. As you can observe from the behavior of drug addicts, the influence of external substances on the internal structure of the human body can have a tremendous impact on behavioral functioning. A disease results when there are changes in the normal cellular mechanisms that affect or control behavior.

Nothing remains stagnant in life and change is inevitable. Likewise, the human body changes everyday and many of the changes can have a direct effect on behavior. It is quite amazing that our bodies can transform over decades as well as during the course of an acute experience without you noticing the transformation. A simple everyday process that is undetected is the sloughing off of epithelial cells. In other words, the dead skin or "ash" is nothing but new skin regenerating. No matter if the changes occur over a long-term period or a short-term period, these transformational changes occur to adapt us to the world we are living.

We discussed in Chapter 6 how addictive-type personalities can be created. Clearly, people can be stressed by society and subsequently develop the need to explore ways to deal with the stresses of life. It is unfortunate, but some people will consume recreational drugs to help them adapt to their surroundings. Besides dealing with the stress of life, drugs can also be used to explore new and "thrilling" ways to occupy one's precious time. Initially, the drug taking behavior may have been for the thrill, but the undetected transformational changes can cause a devastating effect on the entire nervous system. Any change in the nervous system will alter behavior and the person can become dependent on the drug in order for the nervous system to function normally. It is no longer a cheap thrill, but an expensive habit because more and more of the drug is needed to help maintain the imbalanced created by the drug. This is a serious predicament because the quest of the addict is to pursue the feeling that was obtained from that first hit. Crack cocaine, for example, is so potent after one hit that it will cause the drug taker to forever seek the same feeling that was generated from that first high. Unfortunately, the feeling from the initial high will never be obtained, so the drug taker will be sent into a perpetual frenzy to seek that unobtainable feeling. The transformation is deadly and the disease state has thus begun.

No one wants the stigma of a disease to be attached to their behavior. However, the physical state of a drug addict is actually a transformational change in the internal structure that causes their brain to function in an abnormal manner. No matter how much some drug addicts may try to abstain from a substance such as crack cocaine or methamphetamine, the physical changes in the brain from drug abuse are so tremendous that the person might kill to obtain the effect of the drug again. Any substance that could make one kill another person just to obtain the drug has created a diseased state of the mind.

The brain is very responsive to external stimuli, and melinated cells are highly reactive to drugs and other foreign agents that can enter the brain. One of the functions of melanin is to neutralize toxic substances, and it is commonly understood that free radicals are absorbed by melinated cells to provide protection from the damage that can be produced by free radicals. The protective capabilities of melanin can absorb the harmful chemicals and prevent widespread brain damage. I have emphasized transformational changes in this chapter because neuromelanin has the capacity to enhance or negatively affect behavior. The enhancement of neuromelanin containing cells could help to facilitate the conduction of nerve impulses (Moore, 1995). Conversely, a behavioral impairment could occur if neuromelinated cells are overwhelmed with toxic substances (Barnes, 1988). Essentially, drugs can cause transformational changes in the brain and melanin can amplify these changes.

As we learn new things daily, the brain undergoes multiple changes to adapt to the acquisition of new information. The term "plasticity" refers to the brain's ability to form new neural connections for the acquired information. Neural connections can be transformed in response to stimuli that is learned or from external substances such as drugs. Moreover, melinated brain cells can affect transformational changes in the brain, and these pigmented brain cells are highly responsive to drugs. Any structural change in brain cells (specifically melinated cells) can lead to a diseased state. The outcome would be the development of abnormal behavior. For example, Parkinson's Disease is the result of deteriorated pigment cells in the substantia nigra located in the midbrain. The etiology of Parkinson's Disease is unknown, but there is a high probability that some external substance destroys neuromelanin cells in the midbrain. Patients with Parkinson's Disease have impaired motor functioning and they may also experience mood changes such as depression. Even with normal aging, pigmented brain cells lose their protective capabilities and no longer function properly. The combination of normal aging and the accumulation of toxic substances can lead to a diseased state and a deadly transformation in the brain.

THE PHYSIOLOGY OF CRAVING

Every single thought in your mind is a result of electrical activity and chemical communication. In other words, preceding and proceeding every thought depends on the activation of chemicals in the brain. The chemical reactions in the brain are generally classified as neurotransmission. To crave for a drug is to have a specific activation of neurotransmitters that are stimulated by both internal and external factors. When discussing drug addiction, it is important to mention that use and drug abuse are governed jointly by the biochemical properties of a drug, the environment, and personality factors. Therefore, the euphoria associated with the drug effects, the setting in which the drugs are consumed and the type of emotions exhibited by the individual can combine to create a craving for drugs..

In recent years, research has focused on attempts to determine what motivates people to use drugs rather than merely on the effects of drugs. This is an important point because if you can eliminate the desire to consume drugs, you can subsequently decrease drug use and abuse. To the contrary, there are effective tactics that can be used to enhance a craving for drugs with sex and power as motivating factors. The use of sex to sell alcohol to the youth (Moore, Taylor and Turner, 1998), and specifically 40 ounces of malt liquor (Powell, 1995), are perfect examples of the manipulative ways cravings for a drug can be developed.

As mentioned in Chapter 6, creating an addictive-type personality is big business. In contrast to treatment models for addiction (e.g., methadone treatment for opiate abuse), understanding the motivations or cravings for drugs can lead to more effective prevention models for drug abuse (Center for Substance Abuse Prevention, 1993; Moore, 1997). Many drugs are powerful reinforcers and they have a strong biological underpinning. Pleasure seeking for the reinforcing properties of drugs must be prevented to effectively eliminate the physiological craving for drugs. Although I have discussed health activism as a drug prevention model (Moore, 1997), treatment for drug addiction is much more difficult to address.

How can one's body yearn for an external substance rather than depend on the chemicals that already exist in the body? First of all, miseducation about the body being a person's temple is the first problem that could lead a person to seek external substances for the purpose of obtaining a state of euphoria. If you do not respect your own body, then it is easy to neglect it and harm it with foreign substances. The devastating aspect of this circumstance is the fact that a person can become dependent on this foreign substance for normal functioning.

A grip is a firm hold on a particular substance. As we will discuss in the next chapter, the functional properties of melanin can create a grip on a foreign substance and cause a person to be dependent on that substance. In brief, melanin is a biological entity that can hold a drug or substance for a lengthy period of time and cause the brain to change. What occurs is a serious dependence on the drug for the brain to reach a normal state of functioning. What can actually happen is that melanin can absorb certain drugs and set in motion a craving need for the drug. The craving is actually a transformational change in the brain, and the addict is then locked into a perpetual search to obtain another high.

THROWING AWAY THE LOCK AND KEY

If you throw away the lock and key you are assumed to be trapped in prison forever. In terms of drug addiction, I am suggesting that the physical changes caused by consuming drugs can transform the brain and lead to a hopeless chance to fully recover from drug addiction. It is quite obvious that people can overcome drug addiction, but the diseased state created by the addiction can manifest again if the right conditions are created. Those conditions could be related to the environment one is in and/or personality factors.

The severity of drug addiction in today's society has reached epidemic proportions, and it appears as though there are no effective treatments insight. Without a lock (receptor) and key (chemical) suggests that there is no hope for millions of drug addicts. By thinking of addiction as a disease, you can understand why it is assumed that there is no outlet for the addict. Although it is quite obvious that some people can overcome drug addiction and that prevention models can be effective, I am emphasizing the diseased state that may create a hopeless situation toward a real recovery.

The euphoric experience from certain drugs can lead to a perpetual dependence on the drug. Actually, it is the feeling from the drug that keeps the addict perpetually locked into a cell of false euphoria. People are always searching for an external entity to make them feel good; therefore, a culture of drug use is created and poor people with limited outlets are seduced into drug use and abuse. As a society, African Americans are associated with drugs and the color of one's skin has a lot to do with the perceptions about drug use and abuse. For many African Americans, throwing away the lock and key results from a society with no real plan to release people from the confines of drug addiction.

The lock and key in this analysis are respectively the receptor and the specific chemical in the brain that are affected by the drug. Chemicals and receptors are the essential components involved in neurotransmission, and any interference with chemicals and receptors in the brain can excite or inhibit communication in the nervous system. For example, the nervous system requires both electrical and chemical information to function. The electrical communication would utilize charged particles called ions ($K+$, $Na+$, $Ca+$, $Cl-$) to excite or inhibit brain cells. Positively charged ions might stimulate a cell to transmit information whereas negatively charged ions might inhibit a cell's ability to communicate. The electrical activity in the nervous system is important because it can ultimately influence the amount of neurochemicals that are functioning in the brain. Moreover, the brain receptors would be altered because the receptors are dependent upon endogenous chemicals to function properly. Throwing away the lock and key would suggest that the internal imbalance caused by drug consumption may lead to permanent changes in the nervous system.

In the next chapter, we will describe how the physical properties of melanin can attribute to the development of drug addiction. The first African-centered scientific perspective on melanin's role in addiction was made by Carol Barnes (1988). Barnes discussed the harmful effect of toxic drugs on melanin centers within the Black human over a decade ago. He provided supportive evidence that melanin in the Black human is the central reason why he/she becomes addicted quicker and remains addicted longer to drugs.

It is quite obvious why the white scientific establishment would not support such a connection, but the perspective originally presented by Barnes can no longer be overlooked in the African-American community (Newton, 1993). In 1993, Dr. Patricia Newton, an African American psychiatrist, wrote an informative article on drug abuse and addiction with melanin as the central theme. The role of melanin and melanogenesis in the consideration of biological vulnerability in alcohol and other drugs of abuse were considered. Drug abuse and addiction are too prevalent in the African American community for any connection to be overlooked. To extend the ideas of Barnes and Newton, we will explore the physical properties of melanin and how the science of melanin can attribute to addiction.

Chapter 8

Melanin and Drug Binding

In this Chapter, we will present evidence that darkly pigmented cells in both the brain and the body can dramatically influence the behavioral effects of drugs. We will provide evidence that dark does matter in biology, and it is the pigmented cells that can attract certain chemical substances and lead to pathobiochemical processes (Borovansky, 1996). Melanin is not the sole reason for how drug addiction can develop into a diseased state, but it can certainly affect the severity of drug addiction.

Our investigation into melanin's role in drug addiction may imply that there is only a biological model that can be explained. Our emphasis is certainly on biology, but there are other factors that can attribute to addiction. Some models may be biological, environmental or cognitive in their approach. Although most of the current models may focus on an interaction of several factors, we will focus on the biochemical factors related to melanin and drug binding. It is the protective capabilities as a neutralizer of toxic substances that will be discussed in this chapter.

Drug binding to melanin is no longer a speculative phenomena. Scientists have begun to use high tech instruments to harness melanin's natural technological features. In the laboratory, scientists can use chromatography and spectroscopy instrumentation to detect melanin or the binding of drugs to melanin (Howells, Godfrey and Sauer, 1994; Radwanska, Frcackowiak, Ibrahim, Aubry and Kaliszan, 1995; Ibrahim and Aubry, 1995). Since melanin can act as an attractant or reservoir for certain chemicals, synthetic melanin's have been used to detect melanin's binding capacity for certain drugs. Radwanska et al. (1995) used a high performance liquid chromatographic column packed with a stationary phase obtained by chemical immobilization of synthetic L-dopa melanin on silica particles. They were able to predict the potential toxicity of 13 phenothiazine neuroleptics and 2 dibenzapine thymoleptics. By virtue of its binding kinetics, high capacity and mechanical robustness, synthetic melanin offers potential for use in chromatography or solid-phase extraction and may additionally enable modeling of drug-melanin interactions (Howells et al., 1994).

MELANIN TOXICITY

There is substantial evidence that certain drugs and other chemicals are bound to melanin and retained in pigmented cells for long periods of time (Larsson, 1993). The evidence expands over three decades so the topic can be thoroughly investigated. What is emphasized in this chapter is that melanin can bind dangerous chemicals and cause adverse reactions (Larsson, 1993; Lindquist, 1973). Although melanin may be functioning naturally as a protective element, the long-term effects of continuous exposure to dangerous chemicals can destroy the cells containing melanin.

Any internal or external location of the body where the brown to black pigment is found is a potential site for a melanin-drug interaction. Extensive accumulation of drugs by melanin appears to be the most important factor governing the long-term therapeutic/toxicological activities (Salazar-Bookaman, Wainer and Patil, 1994). According to these authors, drugs crossing placental circulation are localized in the mouse fetal eye, a site with a high concentration of melanin. Thus, drugs exhibit a high binding capacity for melanin containing tissues. Studies on synthetic melanin and melanin granules also indicated a high binding capacity of many therapeutic classes of drugs, including psychotropic drugs which are used for treating mental disorders. Chlorpromazine, for example, is used to treat schizophrenia and it has a higher binding capacity than similarly structured compounds. In addition to the liposoluble property of melanin, there is a definite relationship between chemical structure and the affinity of drugs for melanin (Salazar-Bookaman et al. 1994).

There are extensive examples of drug-melanin interactions that can be presented. For example, antimalarial drugs have an affinity for melanin. As we know, the sickle cell gene was an evolutionary response to protect people of African descent from malaria. For those whom did not carry the sickle cell gene, antimalarial drugs such as chloroquine were developed. Chloroquine is also used for the treatment of rheumatoid arthritis. Chloroquine may be a very functional compound to treat some health disorders, but it can induce lesions in the retinal pigment epithelium (Larsson, 1993). These lesions are called retinopathies and the neuroleptic drug chlorpromazine can also induce similar eye lesions. Neuroleptics are used to treat the mental state of psychotic patients suffering from disorders like schizophrenia. Neuroleptics and antimalarial drugs were certainly created for separate health problems, but they can both create lesions in the melinated layer of cells in the eye and lead to blindness.

The eye is located externally in the body and is vulnerable to injury and exposure to toxic environmental insults (Eves et al., 1999). The eye is second only to the liver in showing manifestations of drug toxicity (Tripathi and Tripathi, 1986). There are several populations of pigmented cells in the eye: iris pigment epithelium; ciliary and retinal pigment epithelium; and iridial, ciliary and choroidal melanocytes. It has been suggested that melanin has a protective role and also acts as a biochemical dustbin, mopping up free radicals and other potentially toxic agents (Proctor et al., 1974). Such properties would be important in protecting the eye from the natural toxins of light, oxygen species (including free radicals), in addition to man-made toxins in the form of drugs and industrial chemicals (Eves et al., 1999).

In 1973, Lindquist reported that quinine may induce lesions in the pigmented tissues of the inner ear. The accumulation of quinine in the stria vascularis of the cochlea may cause local degeneration in pigment granules and secondarily cause lesions in the hair cells. The adverse effect is impaired hearing.

Thioureylenes are used as antithyroid drugs. It has been reported (Larsson, 1993) that intake of thioureylenes are incorporated as false precursors into melanin during its synthesis. As a result, this intake can affect melanin synthesis in the melanocytes in the skin and cause a toxic reaction. Since skin melanin is the most visible form of melanin, we need to understand the impact of skin color and drug addiction.

There are mainly two kinds of melanin, the black-brown eumelanin and the yellow-red pheomelanin. In the epidermis of human skin and in the hair, especially in people of African descent, the major part of the pigment consists of eumelanin. In humans with red hair, pheomelanin is the major pigment. Eumelanin and pheomelanin can be mixed in various proportions to create the range of other humans, but it is eumelanin which has received the most attention in drug studies. Mars and Larsson (1999) have demonstrated in an animal model that chloroquine, chlorpromazine, chlomipramine, paraquat, acridine orange, and nickel, which are bound to eumelanin, also bind to synthetic pheomelanin. The binding to pheomelanin, however, is lower. This finding can suggest that the toxicological risks of melanin-related adverse effects are applicable to various skin tones in humans.

Related to skin melanin, vitiligo is a common dermatological disorder characterized by the development of complete pigment loss from focal lesions that tend to increase in size over time. It was first described in 1939 (Oliver et al.) that phenolic compounds could cause cutaneous depigmentation found in vitiligo. According toYang and Boissy (1999), it has been corroborated that various phenols such as 4(para)-tertiary butylphenol (4-TBP), 4-tertiary amylphenol, 4-tertiary butylcatechol (4-TBC) and 2,4-ditertiary butylphenol (DTBP), could induce depigmentation that is clinically and histopathologically indistinguishable from idiopathic vitiligo. It has been proposed that phenolic derivatives compete with tyrosine for hydroxylation by tyrosinase and interfere with the completion of melanin synthesis. Yang and Boissy (1999) demonstrated that 4-TBP competitively inhibited tyrosine hydroxylase.

In general, toxic accumulation of external substances can settle in darkly pigmented brain cells (i.e., neuromelanin). We will discuss neuromelanin in Chapter 8, but it is important to mention here that melanin toxicity can affect the brain. For instance, the nerve cells of the extrapyramidal system contain neuromelanin and the melanin affinity of certain neurotoxic agents may impair movement. 1-methyl-4-phenyl-1,2,3,6-tetrahydropyridine (MPTP) may be involved in the development of damage similar to Parkinson's Disease (Lindquist, Larsson and Lyden-Sokolowski, 1987). Interestingly, the neuroleptics that are used for Schizophrenia can also cause movement problems that look very similar to Parkinson's Disease. The common feature of MPTP and neuroleptics are that they affect the neurotransmitter called dopamine.

Essentially, too much dopamine can cause Schizophrenia and too little dopamine in a specific brain region can cause Parkinson's Disease. Many neurotransmitters such as dopamine are colocalized with neuromelanin. If neuromelanin accumulates toxic substances, then the concentration of dopamine in the affected area is also disturbed. Interfering with the internal balance of dopamine levels can dramatically alter behavior.

Human behavior is not dependent on only one chemical or brain area to function properly, however. Our brains process information via circuits. For dopamine, there are actually two circuits or pathways that produce dopamine: the mesolimbic pathway and the nigrostriatal pathway. The former is more involved in mood disorders linked to Schizophrenia and the latter is involved in movement disorders linked to Parkinson's Disease. In the next section, we will link dopamine to another toxic drug, cocaine.

MELANIN AND COCAINE

There are a multitude of drugs that can bind to melanin, but I have chosen to highlight the effects of cocaine because of its addictive properties. The consumption of cocaine may differentially activate brain circuits containing dopamine. It is postulated (Volkow, Ding, Fowler and Wang, 1996) that periodic and frequent stimulation of the dopaminergic system by cocaine perpetuates the compulsive administration of the drug and the intense craving experienced by cocaine abusers. Continued use and abuse of cocaine can lead to persistent neurological/ psychiatric impairments (Majewska, 1996). The diseased state discussed in Chapter 7 may be due to the possible neuronal degeneration associated with chronic drug abuse.

Some impairments resulting from cocaine toxicity include multi-focal and global ischemia, cerebral ischemia, cerebral hemorrhages, infarctions, optic neuropathy, cerebral atrophy, cognitive impairments, and mood and movement disorders (Majewska, 1996). The utilization of Positron Emission Tomography (PET) has demonstrated that the fast uptake and clearance of cocaine from the brain differs from the pharmacokinetics of other drugs (Volkow, 1996). The fast action of cocaine on the reward centers in the brain make it a very potent substance. The potency of crack cocaine versus cocaine hydrochloride has been questioned, and many people in the African American community believe crack cocaine has been targeted to low income communities. Crack cocaine is thought to be more addictive than its hydrochloride form. In fact, there are even more stringent laws against crack cocaine possession versus cocaine hydrochloride. However, research has provided evidence that the physiological and psychoactive effects of cocaine are similar regardless of whether it is in the form of cocaine hydrochloride or crack cocaine (Hatsukami and Fischman, 1996).

The physiological effects of cocaine on the brain are very important to understand. The most basic reason for making the connection between cocaine and melanin is the common biosynthesis of the two biological substances. Dopamine, for example, is the central biochemical that links cocaine and melanin. Dopamine is a neurotransmitter in the brain that is important for normal behavioral functioning. Fig. 5 describes the main two dopamine pathways in the brain. Some have proposed that it is one of the precursor molecules leading to neuromelanin formation. Since neuromelanin and dopamine coexist in darkly pigmented brain areas in the midbrain (e.g., substantia nigra), it is assumed that neuromelanin is an end-product of neurotransmission involving dopamine.

The amino acid, tyrosine, is another precursor molecule that links dopamine and melanin. There are two enzymes that can convert tyrosine into either dopamine or melanin. Tyrosine hydroxylase can convert tyrosine to eventually form dopamine in the brain and tyrosinase can convert an altered form of dopamine to synthesize melanin in our skin. Understanding this connection makes it quite apparent that a person's overall genetic capacity to produce melanin can attribute to the toxic effects of some drugs.

Any elevation in brain dopamine can increase mood and enhance movement. Furthermore, dopamine is highly associated with the reinforcing properties of psychostimulants such as cocaine and amphetamine. The reinforcing properties are what lead to drug addiction, so it is very important to understand the biochemical effects of cocaine on dopamine.

Cocaine will cause dopamine to remain in the nervous system for a longer period of time and induce a euphoric response (see Fig. 6). The psychopharmacological effects of cocaine require a basic understanding of neurotransmission. First, there is the presynaptic terminal that releases a neurochemical like dopamine. Secondly, the release is into a gap called the synaptic cleft. Thirdly, the neurochemical travels across the synaptic cleft to excite receptors on the postsynaptic terminal. Fourthly, activation of brain receptors stimulates a cascade of biochemical processes that stimulate the brain for action. There are also autoreceptors on the presynaptic terminal and this is where cocaine can exert its primary effect. Cocaine inhibition of dopamine reuptake at the level of the presynaptic terminal has been shown to be the primary biochemical influence on the reinforcing effects of cocaine (Ritz, 1999).

The increased cocaine in the synaptic cleft has several effects that can cause long-term transformational changes in the brain. First, it decreases the synthesis of dopamine by a feedback mechanism. Secondly, dopamine in the synaptic cleft acts via D2 autoreceptors to inhibit the subsequent firing of the presynaptic dopaminergic neuron. Thirdly, the facilitation of dopaminergic neurotransmission results in decreases in postsynaptic neuronal firing. The compounded effect from these transformational changes in the brain are devastating because overtime less dopamine will be synthesized and released.

Ironically, cocaine inhibition of dopamine reuptake is no longer as effective in producing the original drug effects. Although a dopamine deficiency is found in both chronic cocaine abusers and Parkinson's Disease, chronic cocaine abuse does not cause Parkinsonism (Dhopesh, Yagnik and Weddington, 1997).

The inhibition of cocaine reuptake mentioned by Ritz (1999) occurs at a carrier protein on the presynaptic terminal called the dopamine transporter DAT (Volkow et al., 1996; Kiyatkin, 1994; Thibaut, Vaugeois and Petit, 1995). Analysis of the behavior of cocaine in the human brain with PET revealed that cocaine has a strong affinity for the DAT (Volkow et al., 1996). The brain areas involved would be related to the mesolimbic pathway. Since a large body of neuropharmacological evidence suggest that the mesolimbic dopamine system has exclusive importance for the development and maintenance of cocaine addictive behavior, and cocaine is known to interfere in activity of this brain system, examination of mesolimbic dopamine neurons during cocaine self-administration behavior may provide some clues for understanding the drug's addictive properties and regulation of this maladaptive behavior (Kiyatkin, 1994).

It is commonly understood that DAT transports dopamine across the presynaptic membrane. The DAT terminates the action of dopamine in the synapse via reuptake and thus regulates dopamine neurotransmission. The transporter has been studied by direct binding techniques using a variety of ligands which are inhibitors to dopamine transport (e.g., cocaine). Interestingly, cocaine has binding sites on the carrier protein which may be distinct from dopamine binding sites. The DAT gene is also an important candidate gene for psychiatric diseases such as schizophrenia and cocaine abuse (Thibaut et al., 1995). Since the transport of chemicals into the brain is a key function to a drug's potency and effectiveness, it is easily understood how melanin can affect drug binding.

THE BARNES HYPOTHESIS

As an organic chemist, Carol Barnes (1988) was one of the first African-centered scientists to make a connection between melanin and cocaine toxicity. His explanation is very clear and he used an organic analysis to describe how melanin can attribute to drug addiction. In review, he begins with structural similarities between dopamine, melanin and cocaine. Benzene, for example, is a major component of unleaded gasoline. Benzene, aromatic and catechol nucleus are synonymous terms. This structure is also a component of amino acids used by the body. The amino acids can polymerize into neurotransmitters as well as melanin. Therefore, any chemical species that contains the benzene group within its structure will have an attraction for melanin.

Cocaine is a toxic drug and it is attracted to melanin. When the two mix, a new chemical hybrid can be created that can lead to harmful brain effects. During cocaine intoxication, certain neurotransmitters (e.g., dopamine) are depleted from the body. The body will try to use cocaine to do the job for dopamine because cocaine has a similar structure to dopamine. Some neuro-transmitters are also major components of the melanin molecule which means cocaine will blend with melanin and affect multiple neurotransmitter systems.

The function of melanin is for life-promotion and life-protection. However, melanin is degraded and destroyed when highly reactive free radicals are formed in the brain from toxic drugs. As a result, organs with melanin may suffer due to a lack of the necessary concentration of melanin needed to promote vital "life" mechanisms.

When the body has completely used up cocaine and it realizes that dopamine is not available for regular metabolism, it triggers a craving for the drug. The brain has been tricked into thinking that the cocaine chemical is dopamine due to the similarities in chemical structure. According to Barnes, a toxic chemical like cocaine has the potential to co-polymerize into the melanin structure. Once the reaction is complete and the molecule becomes stable, it may remain intact in various melanin centers throughout the body for months

(Ings, 1984; Baweja et al., 1977; Patil, 1972). A significant event such as stress, poor diet, exposure to energy sources, or just normal body requirements, may trigger the melanin molecule to release the stored cocaine into the blood or other reactive channels in the body. The fluctuating release of stored cocaine in the body is uncontrolled by the individual. A large enough dose from this delayed release, therefore, could cause a mental "trip", seizures or even sudden death.

Barnes further hypothesized that serotonin and melatonin are other neurotransmitter systems that can differentially affect people of African descent. Serotonin and melatonin are indoleamines or alkaloids produced in the pineal gland. Many alkaloids are of plant origin and alkaloids in both the body and in nature can have similar structures. For example, the structure of serotonin and hallucinogenic drugs such as LSD, mescaline, psilocin, psilocybin are very similar. Moreover, beta carbolines are natural alkaloids that are produced by the pineal gland via melatonin (Airaksinen, 1981). These products are highly hallucinogenic and are believed to cause "out-of-the-body-experiences", religious trances, etc. According to Barnes this needs further attention because beta carbolines may bind to melanin and produce the psychoactive (magical) effects that are predominate in Black society and culture.

MELANIN AND HAIR

Hair is an obvious site for the colorful expression of melanin. Different colors of hair are a direct result of one's genetic capacity to produce melanin. Interestingly, hair samples are often used for drug testing, and it can be controversial if the test is not sensitive enough to account for the absorptive properties of melanin. In other words, many errors and false accusations in drug testing may actually result from the content of melanin in the hair sample. In fact, it is the binding capacity of melanin to numerous compounds that may appear as though the person with dark hair has been taking drugs.

The color of hair and wool in mammals and feathers in birds is mostly determined by the quantity and quality of melanins that are synthesized in follicular melanocytes and transferred to keratinocytes (Ozeki, Ito and Wkamatsu, 1996). The higher the levels of melanin contained in melanocytes will affect the content of melanin in the hair. People with dark pigmentation should absorb more chemicals from the higher content of melanin in both the skin and the hair.

During melanogenesis or the conversion of tyrosine into eumelanin and pheomelanin, several different enzymes are used and numerous oxidative products are formed. The formation of the black to brown eumelanins follows a slightly different biochemical conversion than pheomelanin. Eumelanin, in contrast to pheomelanin, is converted into 5,6-dihydroxyindole-2-carboxylic acid (DHICA) to form the final step in the biosynthesis of the dark pigment. There are specific laboratory techniques that can be used to analyze these products and to determine which type of melanin is active. High performance liquid chromatography and spectro-photometry are two methods that can be used to analyze the type of pigment in melinated samples.

Ozeki et al. (1996) applied these methods to examine melanins in sheep wool, human hair of various colors and mouse melanin. Although people of African descent were not used for this extensive experiment, it should be noted that dark hair did have a different biochemical expression when compared to light hair. Black wool in Asiatic sheep contains eumelanin with the DHICA content similar to black mouse melanin, while black to brown melanins from human hair contain much lower ratios of DHICA-derived units. Dark brown to brown hair in human contains eumelanin whose chemical properties are indistinguishable from those of black hair. In contrast, light brown, blonde, and red hairs contained pheomelanic pigments with a different proportion of oxidative products.

The same techniques were compared in mammalian eumelanins from hair and melanoma cells (Wilcek, Kondoh and Mishima, 1996). They found that DHICA-derived units in hair and melanoma cells were much higher in rodent pigments (58.8%-98.3%; two species, mouse and hamster were examined) as compared to human eumelanins (19.2%-41.8%; one Caucasian and one Oriental individual were examined). Again, no people of African descent were compared in this study.

From the above data, we can make the connection that the content of melanin in the hair can have properties that may influence drug binding. In a study by Joseph, Su and Cone (1996), cocaine binding to Caucasoid and Africoid hair was studied to demonstrate that the amount and type of melanin present are major factors in determining how much drug enters hair after exposure. They used *in vitro* binding techniques to evaluate the binding of radiolabeled cocaine to different types of treated and untreated hair specimens. Divided male and female Caucasoid (black/brown and blond colored) and Africoid (black colored) hair specimens were extracted to remove lipid components (lipid-extracted hair). Cocaine binding was significantly higher to male Africoid hair compared with other groups. The amount of drug binding was similar among female Africoid and male and female, black/brown Caucasoid specimens. The lowest amount of binding was observed with blond, female Caucasoid specimens. Overall, these experiments suggested that lipids in hair play a minor role in drug binding, whereas melanin functions as a major binding site for cocaine. Natural (ethnic) or artificial (bleaching) differences in melanin content may determine the extent of cocaine entrapment in hair after drug exposure.

To conclude, we have presented experimental evidence that there is a connection between drug binding and melanin. We presented a plethora of substances that can bind to internal as well as external melinated body sites. It is very important to understand that melanin's ability to neutralize harmful and toxic substances can have pathological consequences. Recreational drug intake is a deliberate behavior and should be avoided, and consuming drugs for medicinal purposes should be regulated. It is impossible to totally avoid melanin toxicity because it can occur passively through the oral route, the nasal passage or via the skin. Toxic substances exist everywhere and melanin has been the body's natural protectant. Mother nature's body guard (melanin) cannot do all of the work alone, so it is imperative that each person take the responsibility and make every attempt to feed the body as much natural ingredients as possible. To prevent melanin toxicity, one should be cognizant of what enters the body.

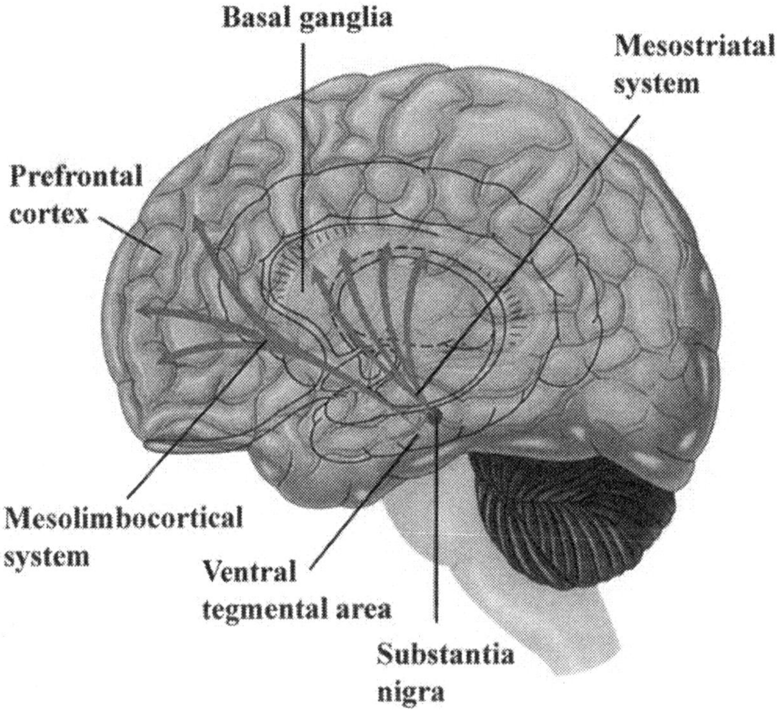

Figure 5 - Two main dopamine pathways: 1) The Mesostriatal system extends from the substantia nigra to the caudate nucleus and it is important for movement; and 2)The Mesolimbocortical system extends from the ventral tegmentum area to the nucleus accumbens and it is associated with pleasure or the reward circuit. Addictive drugs (e.g., cocaine, amphetamine, alcohol and opiates) can turn on the pleasure or reward circuit lying deep within the brain.

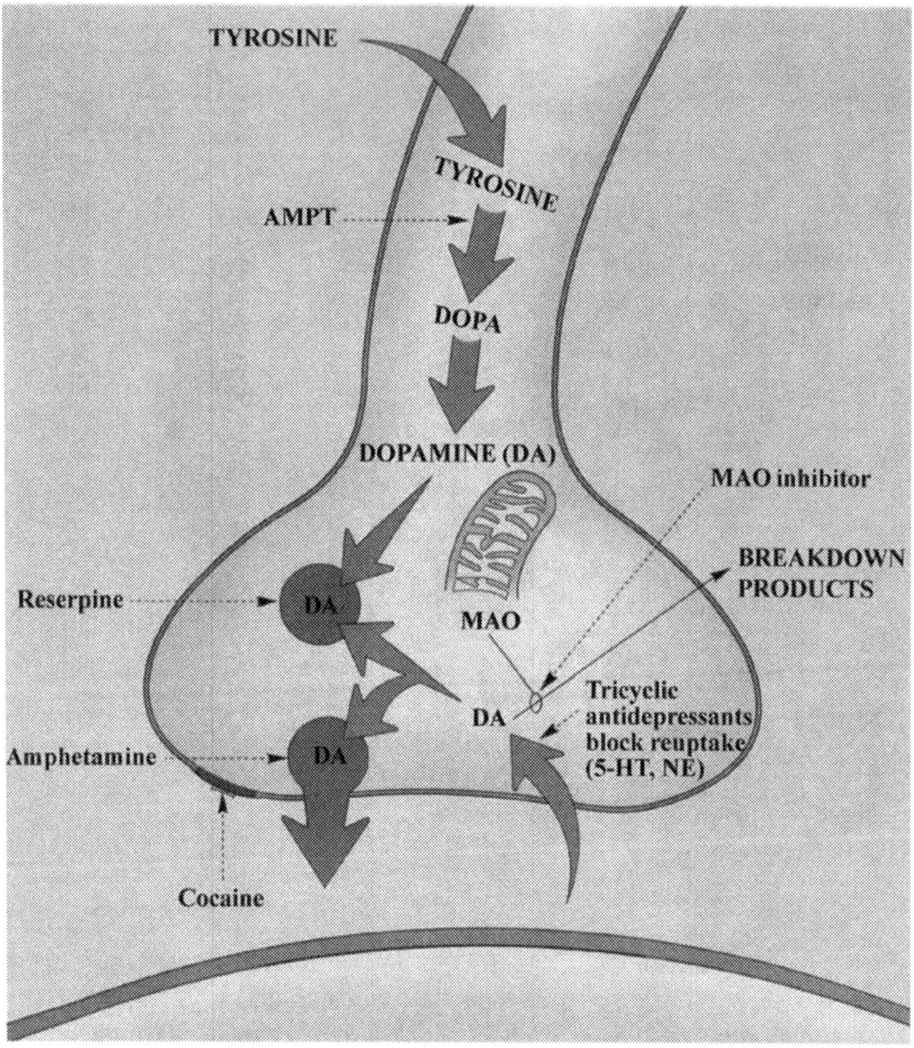

Figure 6 - Mood altering drugs can effect a synapse by blocking the reuptake of neurotransmitters. Melanin in brain cells (i.e., neuromelanin) can enhance these effects by influencing the release of neurotransmitters and strengthen the capability of drugs to bind to receptors.

Chapter 9

An Internal Imbalance

Change is an inevitable part of reality. We grow and develop but we are not ageless wonders. The tick of time moves on and our bodies must adjust and adapt to the harsh environment which surrounds us. Although there is a saying that things get better with time, the aging process actually demonstrates how time can wear the body down. The protective qualities of melanin, however, can help fight against the onslaught of time.

One example of how melanin may be critical for slowing the aging process is the development of weak bones and teeth from poor calcium absorption. Aging can induce an internal imbalance in the bones of many women and resistance to brittle bones may be dependent on a person's genetic capacity to produce melanin. For example, osteoporosis is a common disorder experienced by older white woman. In contrast, African Americans have a lower incidence of fractures than Caucasians (Jacobsen et al., 1990; Farmer et al., 1984; Griffin et al., 1992), which has been attributed to a higher peak bone density in African Americans. It is not clear what factors influence bone loss in African Americans, but several factors have been investigated (Perry et al., 1996). Dietary calcium intake, ethanol intake and endogenous hormone levels have been explored. Perry et al. performed a cross sectional study of bone density, bone composition, demographic variables, bone-related biochemical variables, and hormones likely to affect bone metabolism in African American females from the second to the ninth decades of life. These relationships were compared in a similar group of Caucasian females.

Since melanin is important for the process of calcium absorption for strong bones and teeth, a physiological change due to aging can alter the absorption of calcium. The aging body is unable to process vitamin D synthesis for calcium absorption. Melanin in the skin of darker woman may give them protection from osteoporosis.

Studies that have evaluated mineral metabolism in adult African Americans compared to Caucasians demonstrated significant differences in 25 OHD, a metabolite of vitamin D synthesis (Bell et al., 1985; Gilsanz et al., 1991; Meier, 1991). Therefore, aging may affect the way vitamin D is absorbed in the skin for the utilization of calcium for the bones.

Compared to Caucasian females, African American females have a higher bone density and higher serum estradiol and testosterone levels (Perry et al., 1996). We know there is an external difference in melanin content and this skin differentiation may attribute to the first differences in the incidence of osteoporosis. In addition to melanin's abilities to affect calcium absorption, there are other mechanisms where an internal imbalance can be observed as a result of melanin's biophysical properties.

For example, melanin is able to absorb free radicals and environmental pollutants, and the protective qualities of melanin help to neutralize the damaging effects of molecules on the skin and in the body. Once a chemical is broken down or absorbed by melanin, however, this neutralization can lead to other long-term problems. Moreover, the accumulation of by-products from melanin can present a cascade of negative consequences that can lead to the biological destruction of cells.

It is well understood that one of melanin's functional properties is to act as a neutralizer of harmful free radicals or toxic substances. The biological properties of melanin allow it to absorb, attract and act as a sink for toxic substances. Melanin synthesis can be cytoprotective and accumulate large amounts of melanin within the cell, act as an unstable reservoir for some drugs, and retard the clearance of drugs from the body (Eves et al., 1999). This protective role is a double-edge sword, however, because melanin can also lead to cellular destruction. In other words, melanin can be both life-promoting as well as a sentence for death.

Throughout a person's lifespan, melanin can function as a regulator of what affects the external body as well as what is ingested in the body. It can establish a balanced internal milieu and assist in the maintenance of a healthy life. We eat and digest toxic substances, walk and breathe in pollution and soak in the sun which can destroy our skin. Melanin has a role in protecting us from the substances we digest, the pollutants we ingest, and the ultraviolet radiation we receive from the sun. We can't stop eating, breathing or walking in the sun, but we can be conscious of what we do to our brain/body. Everything you do must be engaged in moderation and not for excess. It is imperative that we not overindulge in the consumption of substances that can be harmful and destructive to our brain/body. Over time, the excessive consumption of toxic substances such as drugs can lead to an imbalanced physical state.

In the case of drug consumption and the subsequent addiction, there is a sequence of events that can lead to both an imbalanced physical and mental state. First, the person must be subliminally seduced (Key, 1973) to create the desire for drugs. Secondly, societal conditions must contribute to the continued use of the drug (Wilson, 1990). Illegal drugs must be made affordable for continued use. Thirdly, the availability of drugs will make it easier for addiction to develop. Ultimately, there will be a transformational change in the body/brain that causes a physical craving for the drug.

An internal imbalance can occur when melanin absorbs too many harmful substances. It can become like a saturated, dirty sponge. For example, it can no longer function to absorb molecules but it can release the toxic chemicals in the brain/body like a dripping sponge full of nasty chemicals. Under normal conditions, melanin can deactivate metabolically excited molecules that can become potentially damaging to cells (McGinness and Proctor, 1973). The absorption and later release of chemicals from melinated cells can lead to an imbalanced state, and the latent release may be triggered by stress. The brain/body, for example, may naturally react to any kind of psychosocial stress by releasing these stored chemicals to cope with the demands of the stressor.

The stable nature of melanin gives it the unique feature to accumulate several biological compounds. For example, various amines, drugs, and a number of metals can be retained in melinated regions of the body for a very long time (Larsson and Tjalve, 1979). Lindquist, Larsson and Lyde-Sokolowski (1987) suggested that melanin's capacity to accumulate and bind a variety of compounds can allow neuromelanin to protect the cells that harbor the pigment by keeping potentially harmful substances bound, and thereafter, slowly releasing the agents in low, non-toxic concentrations. If the brain is saturated and overburdened with these cytotoxic molecules, then behavior is ultimately disturbed. Mental trips that occur months and even years after the consumption of psychedelic drugs such as LSD or PCP are specific examples of how cytotoxic molecules may be slowly released to affect behavior (see Fig. 7).

In sum, the protective role of melanin is to maintain a well-conditioned state of health. It can protect against the numerous chemical and biological agents that exist in our environment, and subsequently eliminate poor health. However, there is always the possibility that melanin might become overprotective. In the case of some neurodegenerative disorders (e.g., Parkinson's Disease), melanin may absorb too much and create a toxic situation (Calne, 1991). Long-term exposure to a toxic compound with high neuromelanin affinity may ultimately cause lesions in the cell (Lindquist et al., 1987).

In sum, melanin can play a significant role in the physiology of drug addiction. From the creation of addictive personalities to the physical properties of melanin, we explored how it does matter to have or not to have melanin. The amount of melanin in the skin as well as in the brain can greatly influence the intensity of some drug effects.

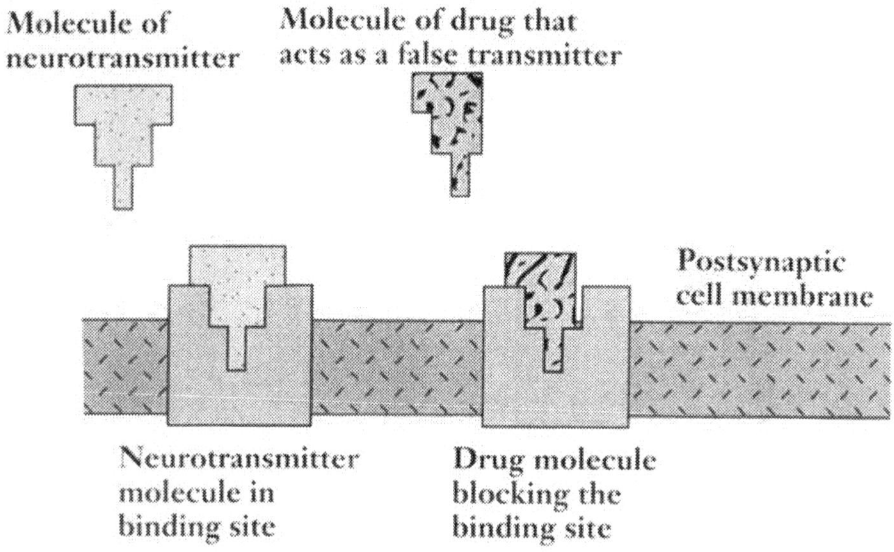

Figure 7 - Drugs have different chemical structures and receptors, and when bound to melanin, a new molecule can form to effect neurotransmission and receptor physiology. In the long-term, drugs bound to melanin can become false transmitters and ultimately affect behavior.

Chapter 10

Dark Secrets Revealed

CHEMICAL WARFARE

It is a sad state of affairs for humanity when the government which supposedly represents you would invest time, money and valuable resources to develop chemicals to kill you. From the AIDS epidemic to the Ebola virus to the current fears about anthrax, the U.S. Government is implicated in the spread of these deadly contagions. With the financial investment in a higher form of killing (Harris and Paxman, 1982), it is quite obvious that the drug crisis is another form of chemical warfare.

Drug trafficking and abuse has crossed all class, race, gender, and national boundaries and is a society-wide and global problem (Lusane, 1991). According to Lusane, what is cast as a "problem" in the white community is, in fact, a crisis in communities of color. Black males particularly young ones, have been trapped in a cycle of poverty and unemployment, nothing less than economic genocide. As a consequence of drug trafficking, we observe the devastating effects of black self-annihilation in service of white domination (Wilson, 1990).

Using drugs to control behavior is one factor that can adversely affect the way a person functions in society. In Chapter 6, we presented the pacification process as a technique to influence the desire and motivation to consume drugs. Although anyone can be exposed to drugs, African American males were the primary focus of the discussion. In a ruling patriarchal society, another male is the greatest threat to the power establishment. Since the U.S.A. is a white male-dominated society, Black males can exhibit a perceived threat to the power elite. The pacification process can explain how the threat can be lessened by involving Black males in an underworld of self-destructive behavior. It is imperative that we reveal the dark secrets that make melanin-dominant individuals vulnerable to the ravaging effects of drugs.

The voluntary consumption of mind-altering drugs is a choice made by the consumer. The initial desire to consume these types of drugs (e.g., methamphetamine, crack cocaine, heroin, marijuana, alcohol) can be instigated externally by forces in society or by internal forces generated in the person's mind. External substances such as recreational drugs are capable of making a person feel good and the consumer has a choice whether or not to consume the drug. The dangerous aspect of experimenting with drugs is the fact that an individual can become involuntarily addicted to a substance. In other words, involuntary addiction is actually drug abuse. This chapter will conclude with recommendations to prevent drug abuse in the African American community by encouraging people to become health activists. Preventing drug abuse is not an easy task; however, we conclude this text with information to educate people on possible ways to prevent drug abuse and to treat those who are affected by the addictive properties of drugs.

ETHNOBIOLOGICAL VULNERABILITY

Issues of biological vulnerability in alcohol and other drug (AOD) abuse for the African American community have been discussed (Newton, 1993). In sum, Newton has provided an informative description of how poor health can lead to addiction:

> "For example, in African American communities there are excessive numbers of fast-food chain outlets whose menus offer an abundance of saturated fats, high cholesterol, and chemical preservatives. This situation, when coupled with the high calorie, high sugar, and high-salt junk foods readily available at the neighborhood and corner stores at low cost, places families in a cycle of licit food chemical addiction that seems to escape the notice of the most conscientious of inhabitants of these areas. The proximity and high number of

> liquor stores, cigarette machines, and over-the-counter single cigarette purchases at these stores, along with "sexy" billboard and magazine advertisements, all serve as strong incentives to addictive behaviors unwittingly sanctioned by the African American community itself. This environment and the licit substances available in it can serve to promote 'addictions' that may, in turn, establish the precursor behavior for addic tion to illicit substances" p. 36.

According to Fig. 8, the dark secret is that the biophysical properties of melanin can bind numerous drugs and differentially affect how a person responds to the toxic effects of drugs. For many African Americans, poor dietary habits and a unique neurochemical system can affect both the physiological and pathophysiological effects of melanin.

The medical-pharmaceutical-industrial complex develops medications for mass distribution. The ethnicity of the consumer is seldom a concern in the developmental phase of designing a new drug. When the new treatments reach the consumer, it is often observed that the expected drug effects do not affect all patients similarly. For instance, the chemical structure of certain drugs and the movement of specific drugs through a person's physiological system can have an impact on a person's behavioral response to a drug. In addition to the potential pharmacokinetic and pharmacodynamic differences, pharmacogenetic factors may have an effect on producing interethnic differences. To reiterate, melanin is a major genetic factor contributing to the differential drug effects that exist between ethnic groups.

Ethnobiological differences in response to drugs have been observed with both psychoactive or mind-altering drugs (Lin, Poland and Chien, 1990; Strickland, Lin, Fu, Anderson and Zheng, 1995; Wood and Zhou, 1991) as well as nonpsychoactive drugs (Flaherty and Meagher, 1980). Strickland and Gray (2000) explored the significance of ethnobiological variation in drug responsivity to drugs that are known to treat mood disorders such as depression, anxiety and schizophrenia. Many of the drugs that have been developed to treat mental disorders affect neurotransmitter systems that come from melinated centers in the brain. For example, norepinephrine, serotonin and dopamine are neurotransmitters involved in mood disorders and each neurochemical is produced from specific brain nuclei that are visibly melinated.

According to Strickland et al. (2000), most comparative studies that have demonstrated pharmacokinetic differences contrasted Asian and Caucasian populations. We cannot overlook the importance of understanding the contrast with African Americans because there are specific genetic differences that can explain the variations in drug effects. Adding African American populations to drug studies is critical since there are documented reports that African Americans are prescribed a greater volume of sedating compounds (Lin, Poland and Lesser, 1986).

The breakdown and/or metabolism of drugs in a person's brain/body is dependent upon enzymes. The differential expression of enzymes is a genetic factor that could determine what type of effect a drug can have on a person's behavior. Humans have genetic polymorphisms for enzymes and this contributes to the variations we are discussing. Genetic polymorphisms in the functional expression of enzymes underlies the well documented interpatient variability (Meyer, Zanger, Grant and Blim, 1990; Pollock, 1994).

For example, most psychotropic agents are metabolized by one of the hepatic cytochrome P-450 isoenzymes. Two of the most often encountered p-450 isoenzymes are the IID6 and the IIC19 (Kalow, 1993). The IID6 isoenzyme is responsible for the metabolism of many tricyclic antidepressants, selective serotonergic reuptake inhibitors and most antipsychotics. While only 2.9% to 10% of European Americans are IID6-mediated "poor metabolizers," a study by Kalow (1993) suggests that as many as 33% of African Americans have a "gene alteration" in this isoenzyme which results in a slower metabolic rate. The IIC19 isoenzyme is involved in the metabolism of diazepam, and the demethylation of the tertiary tricyclic antidepressants (Goldstein, Faletto, Romkes-Sparks et al., 1994). While only 3% of European Americans are IIC19 poor metabolizers, approximately 18%-22% of African Americans are IIC19 poor metabolizers, suggesting a slower rate of metabolism of some benzodiazepines and tertiary tricyclic antidepressants in African Americans. A slower rate of metabolism may attribute to a greater physiological response to the drug.

The different response rates in African American patients is not an infrequent phenomenon. Raskin, Thomas and Crook (1975) used a number of psychometric scales to assess the effects of chlorpromazine and imipramine. In a comparison of 159 African American and 555 European American inpatients, it was observed that African Americans manifest more rapid improvement and African American men were therapeutically more responsive to the antidepressant imipramine. Ziegler, Clayton and Biggs (1977) demonstrated that African American patients had significantly higher (50%) nortriptyline plasma levels compared to European Americans. In a study of indigenous African outpatients from Tanzania, the patients responded to cloimipramine in much lower doses than those recommended in western textbooks (Kilonzo, Kaaya, Rweikiza, Kassam and Moshi, 1994). Although these clinical reports suffer from significant methodological concerns, the data suggest that African Americans treated with tricyclic antidepressants will have higher plasma levels per dose, more side effects with equivalent plasma levels, and earlier onset of action than European Americans (Strickland et al. 2000). Also, differences in diet, possibly from the role of regional differences in fat intake, may contribute to the ethnic differences (Kalow, Goedde and Agarwal, 1986).

ETHNIC SPECIFIC ALCOHOL PRODUCTS

Another dark secret revealed to the Black man is the experience of the Red man with the White man. For example, the indigenous people of this land (commonly called Native Americans) were partially conquered by chemical warfare. Peyote, a hallucinogenic plant, had been used for centuries mainly, but not solely, for religious and spiritual purposes. Natural intoxicants were commonly used by native people, however, the use of peyote and other plants came under attack with the introduction of alcohol. Guns, disease and alcohol were used by White colonialists in the war to conquer lands owned by Native Americans. Researchers believe that while alcoholism among Native Americans was not initially genetic, heredity was a key factor in their susceptibility to addiction (see Mancall, 1995). Historically, alcohol was deadly medicine for Native Americans, and the etiology for alcoholism in the Native American community was linked to an enzyme deficiency that alters the breakdown of alcohol.

Since alcohol decimated the health of a once vibrant people (i.e., Native Americans), a lesson should be learned by African Americans to combat ethnic specific alcohol products. It is interesting to note that many commercialized sporting events have alcohol companies for sponsors. Some of the commercials that are shown during Black-oriented programs have specific types of alcohol commercials (e.g., malt liquor advertisements). As a result of these marketing schemes, any objective observer can randomly select an inner city park and playground and see young African American males who have been seduced to consume malt liquor. Many are consuming malt liquor during and after a basketball game. The consumption of any form of alcohol after a strenuous activity is not healthy. The body needs to be replenished with water and electrolytes. Consuming alcohol after playing basketball can attribute to numerous health risks, stimulate arguments and even lead to death as a result of homicide. Further discussion on the implications of black-on-black violence can be found in other texts (Bulhan, 1985; Wilson, 1990).

Physiologically, there is a severe problem with consuming the different types of alcohol that are marketed to low income African Americans. For example, the cheap wines such as Wild Irish Rose, Madd Dog 20/20 and Thunderbird are potent alcoholic substances that have the words "contains sulfites" on the label. Although other alcoholic beverages and some food items contain sulfites, it is the dangerous levels of sulfites in the aforementioned beverages that can be a problem. Long-term consumption can potentially lead to neuropathological damage. For instance, McDonald and Johnston (1990) have reported on the role of excitatory amino acids (EAAs) in developmental neurologic disorders. In fact, there is a metabolic amino acid disorder called sulfite oxidase deficiency (SOD), and it is fatal in childhood. The disorder is characterized by widespread neuronal injury and destruction, mental retardation and cerobrospinal fluid levels of the EAA L-sulfocysteine (Irreverre, Mudd, Heizer and Laster, 1967). The effects of SOD are indirectly related to our discussion since the effects of high sulfite levels from alcohol consumption may produce similar mental disturbances and neuropathologic damage. Concisely, L-sulfocysteine is not normally present in the human body, and this abnormal metabolite is the result of a deficiency of the enzyme sulfite oxidase in brain and peripheral organs (Mudd, Irreverre and Laster, 1967). Orally consuming sulfites in alcoholic drinks can elevate L-sulfocysteine to dangerous levels and mimic the neuropathological changes associated with SOD. Besides sulfites, consumers would need to ask what other ingredients are in the potent beverages that are marketed directly to African Americans. Many of the ads marketed to African Americans are for the purchase of dark-colored, heavy-bodied distilled alcohol which has a much higher ethanol content than the light-colored distilled alcohol (Goddard, 1993). Malt liquor is much darker than the "light" beer that is directly marketed to White males. African Americans should become wiser consumers and pay more attention to the ingredients of the substances that are purposefully marketed to them.

A shocking example that magnifies the potential danger of ethnic specific alcohol products is how the apartheid regime in South Africa planned to concoct drinks to eliminate Black males in South Africa. A quite disturbing speech by the South African President P.W. Botha was reported in the August 18, 1985 edition of the Sunday Times, a South African Newspaper. President Botha ordered the use of chemicals to be placed in the drinks of Blacks. This former leader of the nation of South Africa stated, "...We should now make use of the chemical weapon...My scientists have come up with a drug that could be smuggled into their brews to effect slow poisoning results and fertility destruction. Working through drinks and manufacturing of soft drinks geared to the Blacks could promote the channels of reducing their population." The apartheid regime has been dismantled, but there are entirely too many similarities between the old USA (United South Africa) and the present U.S.A. We should never forget how the powers that be will do whatever is necessary to maintain power. By any means necessary also means to poison innocent people.

DRUG ABUSE PREVENTION VIA HEALTH ACTIVISM

Our society is in trouble unless we seriously respect the disease state that can be produced by consuming drugs. In this materially-oriented culture, "things" are important. People become secondary to material items. As a result, people become less aware of how to deal with social relationships. Subsequently, it is easy for a dependence to develop on a material item. It is possible to be addicted to people, cars, clothes, books, food and other inanimate items, but our concern is external substances that can be consumed to alter one's mental state. A simple process to avoid the desire to consume unhealthy substances is to develop positive relationships with people. Avoiding contact with people and minimizing the opportunities to converse with people may be the first stage to experimenting with drugs. The drug may fill the void of positive human contact. In African-centered communities, interpersonal relationships are very important for a healthy state of mind. Drug abuse prevention and treatment should focus on therapies that encourage human contact. Interpersonal relationships should be important for all people no matter what culture, but African-centered communities are clearly dependent on the strength of interpersonal relationships.

There are no simple solutions to prevent drug abuse, but promoting a healthy lifestyle can be helpful. The question of alcohol and other drug (AOD) abuse in the African American community has been linked to three processes (Goddard, 1993) that can negatively influence a positive outlook on health. According to Goddard, the primary processes that have an impact on the African American community include economic exploitation, White supremacy (racism), political domination, and psychosocial stress. The second process is the general availability of alcohol and drugs in the African American community. The third process is the impact of the media. To prevent disease and promote health, all of these processes must be addressed by health activists.

Moreover, the promotion of health activism in the African American community requires a sincere commitment to making personal changes in lifestyle. To combat AOD abuse, proper education is needed to guide African Americans away from peer pressure and the intense desire to accumulate material items. Also, an African-centered perspective is needed to educate African American children into a positive way of thinking and viewing the world. Without this focus, by the end of the preschool period (age 5) we can predict with a high degree of accuracy those children that are destined to fail and those that are likely to succeed (Rashid, 1989). Although independent schools can successfully combat the ravages of AOD abuse with positive educational experiences, the masses of African American children are still caught up in a system of public education that is extremely efficient in transmitting poverty and ignorance from one generation to the next. According to Rashid (1989), it is important that African American adults in general, and parents in particular, begin to view themselves as the primary intervening forces in the socialization of young children.

A well structured educational system focusing on the cultural viewpoints of African people is an excellent starting point to socialize African American children. White-produced television programs, distorted images in the media and poor public education are factors that have negatively socialized too many misguided youth. Television, the media, and proper education, however, can also be used as motivating forces to promote and maintain positive health. One suggestion to maintain positive health in the African American community should begin with a study of the historical legacy of enslavement. Racism and the oppression associated with enslavement are very negative phenomena that continue to influence the behavior of African Americans. A serious dialogue pertaining to the lasting effects of enslavement could help to address the poor health status in the African American community.

For instance, the trafficking of human lives took a significant toll on the humanity of African people. The oppression associated with the enslavement process has dramatically influenced the history of African Americans and their perception of reality. For any individual that was previously subjugated, it is easy to dwell on the evils of the enslavement process and to hate those people who initiated the subjugation. However, a holistic world view would not consider evil or suffering as ultimately important. The vital question to liberate the mind, body and spirit is to focus on the source of the evil or the cause of the suffering. Knowing what really happened in the past would assist in moving in a positive direction.

The 1994 full-length docudrama called *Sankofa,* which was written, directed and produced by an African (Haile Gerima), is an excellent resource to begin liberating minds from the horrors of the past. It would not only be healing for people in the African diaspora, it would also be revealing to those who have benefitted from the trafficking of human cargo. *Sankofa* returns the viewer to the experience of slavery, and it can be one of many tools to promote positive mental health in African Americans. The fact that there has been a media white-out on *Sankofa* helps to explain why America is not ready for a serious discourse on race. Although President Bill Clinton established a Race Advisory Board in 1997, there was no discussion of a docudrama called *Sankofa.* Even more glaring is what the succeeding administration did under the leadership of President George W. Bush. The Bush administration chose not to send an official delegation to attend the 2001 World Conference Against Racism and Xenophobia held in South Africa. The blatant and arrogant disregard for sensitive humanitarian issues incited enemies of the U.S.A. to attack the World Trade Center on September 11, 2001, a week after the conference concluded.

The end result of the World Trade Center tragedy reveals that it was a serious matter for a group of people (i.e., Middle Eastern Muslims) to feel neglected on a global scale. In the U.S.A., many African American males have felt neglected, but they have never committed such a horrendous suicidal act. Many African American males in the current generation of youth may feel powerless because too often someone else is defining their reality. As a group of people, African American youth have a serious character problem when the first thought that comes to mind is athlete, criminal or "corner hanger." The glamorization of African American athletes is a classic example of a gross distortion in the reality of the human experience. For grown men to be dressed in outfits and costumes and make exorbitant amounts of money to hop, skip and jump is a serious flaw in the structure of Western society. A man's worth is thus measured in terms of his physical attributes and personal and social relationships with a materialistic world instead of his mental capacity to serve the community. When true manhood is consciously realized, "wealth" is not seen in monetary terms alone. The richness of life is connected with fulfilling one's social, moral and biological obligations. Similar to obtaining true wealth, the maintenance of positive health implies well-being of mind, body and spirit. A responsible wealthy and healthy person should live in harmony with neighbors, the environment and oneself.

In conclusion, one strategy to promote health activism is through the use of seminars and forums. The open dialogue is needed to properly inform African American males of the negative factors associated with AOD abuse. The way drugs and alcohol have been used historically to control social movements and to pacify people can be critical information to thwart the continual consumption of AODs. In addition, an historical analysis of why African Americans consumed pork products like intestines and high salt diets with limited fiber may help to explain the high incidence of cancer, hypertension and heart disease in the African American community. The promotion of health activism will require an educated cadre of committed individuals who will be as committed as civil rights activists.

They will need to initiate an assault on the exploitative media images that may influence African American males to consume unhealthy substances. Moreover, a model of action must come from the lessons of the alternative health movement associated with the Black Consciousness movement of the late 1960s and 1970s (Semmes, 1996). Healthy eating habits, proper diets and nutrition should continue to be popularized in the African American community to optimize healthy lifestyles.

CONCLUSION

War exists in many forms, and the use of drugs to thwart human progress can be considered chemical warfare. The focus of this chemical warfare is not limited to African Americans, but this group is highlighted because they live in the most powerful nation on the planet. The powers that be must do whatever they can to keep the most potential threat to their power in a place of subjugation. As the late John H. Clarke frequently stated, "...powerful people cannot afford to educate powerless people for fear they will ultimately take their power away from them." There is no mystery or secret as to why African Americans are in a state of confusion about their destiny on this planet.

Dark Matters-Dark Secrets was written to revitalize an interest in the history and the heritage of people of African descent. To claim a heritage, one must first know their history. In reality, the European conquest of Black nations has made all of African history a dark secret. Africans who were brought to the Americas were once Kings and Queens like King Akhenaton and Queen Nerfertiti on the front cover of this book, but they have fallen from grace. There are plenty of written reminders in ancient Kemet to prevent a fall from grace, but the current educational system is perfectly planned to disseminate misinformation. The dark secret is not only that melanin can negatively influence the effects of some drugs, but that the history and heritage of melanin-dominant people has become a dark secret that should be revealed. If there is a chance to obtain freedom from the shackles of oppression, then it would begin with unlocking the chains and images of psychological slavery (Akbar, 1984).

In this concluding chapter, we have revealed that drugs have been integral in keeping the physical and mental shackles in place. The link between deadly drugs and African Americans began in the era of the slave trade (Lusane, 1991). If we seriously understood the whole process of extracting a human from their home and culture, physically debilitating them, mentally handicapping them, and spiritually destroying them, it is quite obvious that you would have a dysfunctional and warped reality for generations to come. This is no secret. However, the key to freedom and the answer to genocide faced by people in the African diaspora is in their history and heritage. There is no secret or riddle to what our ancestors wrote on the temples and documents in Kemet - KNOW THYSELF. After centuries of exploitation, it is now time to endarken ourselves in mind, body and consciousness. In the context of the topic of discussion, the modern application of the words of Imhotep should read:
Eat right, stay fit and let almighty RA bathe us with the life force it generates.

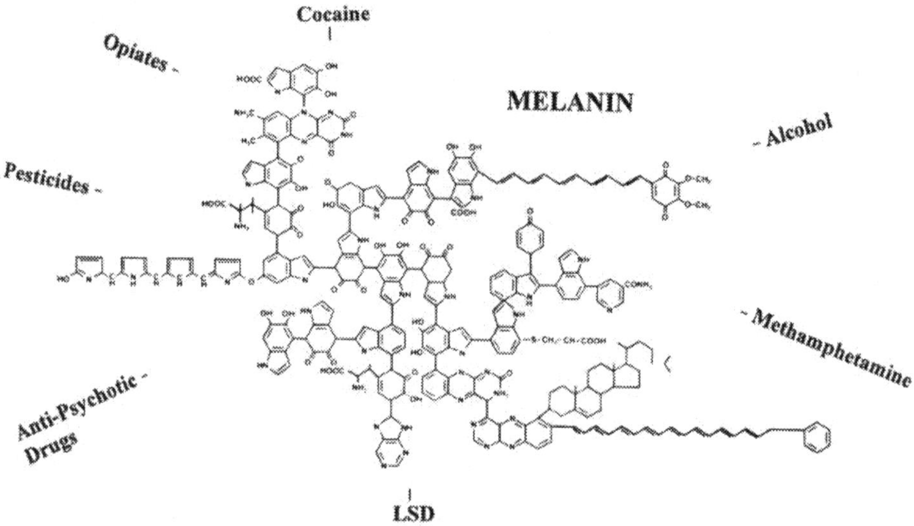

Figure 8 - Melanin is a complex biopolymer, and the binding properties of melanin can attract numerous chemical substances.

REFERENCES

Airaksinen, M.M. and Kari, I. (1981). B-carbolines, psychoactive compounds in the mammalian body. Medical Biology, 59, 21-34.

Akbar, N. (1984). Chains and Images of Psychological Slavery. New Jersey: New Mind Productions

Amen, N.A. (1993). The Ankh: African Origin of Electromagnetism. Jamaica, NY: Nur Ankh Amen Press.

Andrews, M. (1989). Color Me Right...Then Frame Me in Motion. Tennessee: Seymour-Smith, Inc.

Ani, M. (1994). YURUGU: An African-centered Critique of European Thought and Behavior. Trenton, NJ: Africa World Press, Inc.

Barnes, C. (1988). Melanin: The Chemical Key to Black Greatness,Vol.l. Houston, Texas: C.B. Publishers.

Barnes, C. (1993). Jazzy Melanin: A Novel. Houston, Texas: Melanin Technologies.

Baweja, R. et al. (1977). Comparative binding between cocaine and various drugs to synthetic levodopa melanin. Journal of Pharmaceutical Science, 66(11), 1544-1547.

Bell, N.H. et al. (1985). Evidence for alteration of the vitamin D-endocrine system in blacks. Journal of Clinical Investigation, 76, 470-473.

Borovansky, J. (1996). Free radical activity of melanins and related substances: biochemical and pathobiochemical aspects. Sb Lek, 97(1), 49-70.

Bradley, M. (1991). The Iceman Inheritance: Prehistoric Sources of Western Man's Racism, Sexism and Aggression. New York: Kayode Publications Ltd. (originally published 1978).

Bulhan, H. (1985). Frantz fanon and the psychology of oppression. New York: Plenum press.

Bynum, E.B. (1999). African Unconscious: Roots of Ancient Mysticism and Modern Psychology. New York: Teachers College Press.

Calne, D.B. (1991). Neurotoxins and degeneration in the central nervous system. Neurotoxicology, 12, 335-340.

Center for Substance Abuse Prevention (1993). L.L. Goddard (Ed.). An African-centered Model of Prevention for African-American Youth at Risk. CSAP Technical Report 6. Rockville, MD: U.S. Department of Health and Human Services.

Dhopesh, V.P., Yagnik, P.M. and Weddington, W.W. (1997). Can cocaine abuse cause parkinsonism? American Journal of Addiction, 6(2), 177-179.

Eves, P., Smith-Thomas, L., Hedley, S., Wagner, M., Balafa, C. and MacNeil, S. (1999). A comparative study of the pigment on drug toxicity in human choroidal melanocytes and retinal pigment epithelial cells. Pigment Cell Research, 12, 22-35.

Farmer, M.E., White, L.R., Brody, J.A. and Bailey, K.R. (1984). Race and sex differences in hip fracture incidence. American Journal of Public Health, 74, 1374-1380.

Flaherty, J.A. and Meagher, R. (1980). Measuring racial bias in inpatient treatment. American Journal of Psychiatry, 127, 679-682.

Forbes, J. (1992). Columbus and Other Cannibals. New York: Autonomedia.

Gilsanz, V., et al. (1991). Changes in vertebral bone density in black girls and white girls during childhood and puberty. New England Journal of Medicine, 325, 1597-1600.

Goddard, L.L. (1993). Background and scope of the alcohol and other drug problem. In L.L. Goddard (Ed.). An African-centered model of prevention for African-American youth at high risk. (pp. 11-18). Rockville, MD: U.S. Department of Health and Human Services.

Goldstein, J.A., Faletto, M.B., Romkes-Sparks, M. et al. (1994). Evidence that CYP2C19 is the major (S)-mephenytoin 4'-hydroxylase in humans. Biochemistry, 33, 1743-1752.

Griffin, M.R., Ray, W.A., Fought, R.L. and Melton, L.J. III (1992). Black-white differences in fracture rates. American Journal of Epidemiology, 136, 1378-1385.

Harris, R. And Paxman, J. (1982). A Higher Form of Killing: The Secret Story of Chemical and Biological Warfare. New York: The Noonday Press.

Hatsukami, D.K. and Fischman, M.W. (1996). Crack cocaine and cocaine hydrochloride. Are the differences myth or reality. Journal of the American Medical Association, 276(19), 1580-1588.

Howells, L., Godfrey, M. and Sauer, M.J. (1994). Melanin as an adsorbent for drug residues. Analyst, 119(12), 2691-2693.

Ibrahim, H. And Aubry, A.F. (1995). Development of a melanin-based high performance liquid chromatography stationary phase and its use in the study of drug-melanin interactions. Analytical Biochemistry, 229(2), 272-277.

Ings, R.M.J. (1984). The melanin binding of drugs and its implications. Drug Metabolism Reviews, 15(5&6), 1183-1212.

Irreverre, F., Mudd, S.H., Heizer, W.D. & Laster, L. (1967). Sulfite oxidase deficiency. Biochemical Medicine, 1, 187-217.

Jacobson, S.J., et al. (1990). Hip fracture incidence among the old and very old: a population-based study of 745,435 cases. American Journal of Public Health, 80, 871-873.

Joseph, R.E., Su, T.P. and Cone, E.J. (1996). *In vitro* binding studies of drugs to hair: influence of melanin and lipids on cocaine binding to Caucasoid and Africoid hair. Journal of Analytical Toxicology, 20(6), 338-344.

Kalow, W., Goedde, H.W. and Agarwal, D.P. (Eds.)(1986). Ethnic Differences in Reactions to Drugs and Xenobiotics. Proceedings of a meeting held in Titisee, Federal Republic of Germany, October, 1985. New York: Liss.

Kalow, W. (1993). Pharmacogenetics: Its biologic roots and the medical challenge. Clinical Pharmacological Therapeutics, 54, 235-241.

Kambon, K.K. (1998). African/Black Psychology in the American Context: An African-Centered Approach. Tallahassee, FL: Nubian Nation Publications.

Key, W.B. (1973). Subliminal Seduction. New York: Signet.

Kilonzo, G.P., Kaaya, S.F., Rweikiza, J.K., Kassam, M. and Moshi, G. (1994). Determination of appropriate cloimipramine dosage among depressed African outpatients in Dar es Salaam Tanzania. Central African Journal of Medicine, 40(7), 178-182.

King, R. (1990). African Origin of Biological Psychiatry. Tennessee: Seymour-Smith Inc.

King, R. (1994). Melanin: A Key to Freedom. Hampton, VA: U.B. & U.S. Communications Systems, Inc.

Kiyatkin, E.A. (1994). Dopamine mechanisms of cocaine addiction. International Journal of Neuroscience, 78(1-2), 75-101.

Larsson, B. and Tjalve, H. (1979). Studies on the mechanisms of drug-binding to melanin. Biochemical Pharmacology, 28, 1181-1187.

Larsson, B.S. (1993). Interaction between chemicals and melanin. Pigment Cell Research, 6, 127-133.

Lin, K.M., Poland, R.E. and Chien, C.P. (1990). Ethnicity and psychopharmacology: Recent findings and future research directions. In E. Sorel (Ed.), Family, Culture and Psychobiology. New York: Legas.

Lindquist, N.G. (1973). Accumulation of drugs on melanin. Acta Radiologic, Suppl. 325, 1-92.

Lindquist, N.G., Larsson, B.S. and Lyden-Sokolowski, A. (1987). Neuromelanin and its possible protective and destructive properties. Pigment Cell Researc

Lusane, C. (1991). Pipe Dream Blues: Racism and the War on Drugs. Boston, MA: South End Press.

Mahabuti, H.R. (1978). Enemies: Clash of Races. Chicago, IL: Third World Press.

Majewska, M.D. (1996). Cocaine addiction as a neurological disorder: implications for treatment. NIDA Research Monograph, 163, 1-26.

Mancall, .C. (1995). Deadly Medicine: Indians and Alcohol in Early America. Ithaca, NY: Cornell University Press.

Mars, U. and Larsson, B.S. (1999). Pheomelanin as a binding site for drugs and chemicals. Pigment Cell Research, 12, 266-274.

Meier, D.E. et al. (1991). Calcium, vitamin D, and parathyroid hormone status in young white and black women: association with racial differences in bone mass. Journal of Clinical Endocrinology Metabolism, 72, 703-710.

McDonald, J.W. and Johnston, M.V. (1990). Physiological and pathophysiological roles of excitatory amino acids during central nervous system development. Brain Research Reviews, 15, 41-70.

McGinness, J. and Proctor, P. (1973). The importance of the fact that melanin is black Journal of Theoretical Biology, 39, 677-688.

Moore, T.O. (1995). The Science of Melanin: Dispelling the Myths. Silver Spring, MD: Beckham House Publishers.

Moore, T.O. (1997). Historical challenges to maintaining health in African American males. Challenge: A Journal of Research on African American Men, 8 (1), 45-57.

Moore, T.O., Taylor, D. And Turner, D. (1998). African American youth perceptions of alcohol advertisements: A preliminary analysis. Challenge: A Journal of Research on African American Men, 9(2), 67-82.

Mudd, S.H., Irreverre, F. and Laster, L. (1967). Sulfite oxidase deficiency in man: demonstration of the enzymatic defect, Science, 156, 1599- 1602.

Newton, P.A. (1993). Issues of biological vulnerability in AOD for the African American Community. In L.L. Goddard (Ed.). An African-centered Model of Prevention for African-American Youth at High Risk (pp. 35-45). Rockville, MD: U.S. Department of Health and Human Services.

Oliver, E.A., Schwartz, L. and Warren, L.H. (1939). Occupational leucoderma. Journal of theAmerican Association, 113, 927-928.

Ozeki, H., Ito, S. and Wakamatsu, K. (1996). Chemical characterization of melanins in sheep wool and human hair. Pigment Cell Research, 9(51-57).

Patil, P.N. (1972). Cocaine-binding by the pigmented and the non-pigmented iris and its relevance to the mydriatic effect. Investigative Opthalmology, 11(9), 739-746.

Perry, H.M. et al. (1996). Aging and bone metabolism in African American and Caucasian women. Journal of Clinical Endocrinology and Metabolism, 81(3), 1108-1117.

Pollock, B.G. (1994). Recent developments in drug metabolism of relevance to psychiatrists. Harvard Review of Psychiatry, 2, 204-213.

Pookrum, J. (1993). Vitamins and Minerals from A to Z. Brooklyn, NY: A&BBooks Publishers.

Powell, A. (1995). Message in a Bottle: The 40 oz Scandal. Chicago: Renaissance Press.

Proctor, P., McGinness, J. and Corry, P. (1974). A hypothesis on the preferential destruction of melanized tissues. Journal of Theoretical Biology, 48, 19-22.

Radwanska, A, Frcackowiak, Ibrahim, Aubry and Kaliszan (1995).

Chromatographic modelling of interactions between melanin and phenothiazine and dibenzazepine drugs. Biomedical Chromatography, 9(5), 233-237.

Rashid, H.M.. (1989). Divergent paths in the development of African-American males: A qualitative perspective. Urban Review, 12(1),1-13.

Raskin, A., Thomas, H. and Crook, M.A. (1975). Antidepressants in black and white inpatients. Archives in General Psychiatry, 32, 643-649.

Ritz, M.C. (1999). Molecular mechanisms of addictive substances. In R.J. Neisink et al. (Eds.). Drugs of Abuse and Addiction: Neurobehavioral Toxicology (pp. 151-189). Boca Raton, FL: CRC Press.

Salazar-Bookaman, M.M., Wainer, I. and Patil, P.N. (1994). Relevance of drug-melanin interactions to ocular pharmacology and toxicology. Journal of Ocular Pharmacology, 10(1), 217-239.

Semmes, C.E. (1996). Racism, Health and Post-Industrialism: A Theory of African-American Health. Westport, CT: Praeger

Skinner, B.F. (1971). Beyond Freedom and Dignity. New York: Bantam Books.

Strickland, T.L., Lin, K.M., Fu, P., Anderson, D. and Zheng, Y. (1995). Comparison of lithium ratio between African American and Caucasian bipolar patients. Society of Biological Psychiatry, 37, 325-330.

Strickland, T.L. and Gray, G. (2000). Neurobehavioral disorders and pharmacologic Intervention. In E. Fletcher-Janzen, T. Strickland and C.R. Reynolds. Handbook of Cross-Cultural Neuropsychology. pp.

361-369. New York:Kluwer Academic/Plenum Publishers.

Thibaut, F., Vaugeois, J.M. and Petit, M. (1995). The dopamine transporter: characterization and physiologic implications. Encephale, 21(6), 445-451.

Tripathi, R.C. and Tripathi, B.J. (1986). The eye. In H. Riddell (Ed.), Proceedings Pathology of Drug-Induced and Toxic Diseases (pp. 377). New York: Churchill Livingstone.

Volkow, N.D., Ding, Y.S., Fowler, J.S. and Wang, G.J. (1996). Cocaine addiction: hypothesis derived from imaging studies with PET. Journal of Addiction, 15(4), 55-71.

Welsing, F.C. (1991). The Isis Papers: The Keys to the Colors. Chicago: Third World Press.

Wilczek, A., Kondoh, H. and Mishima, Y. (1996). Composition of mammalian eumelanins: analyses of DHICA-derived units in pigments from hair and melanoma cells. Pigment Cell Research, 9, 63-67.

Wilson, A.N. (1990). Black-on-Black Violence: The Psychodynamics of Black Self-Annihilation in Service of White Domination. New York: Afrikan World InfoSystems.

Wood, A.J. and Zhou, H.H. (1991). Ethnic differences in drug disposition and responsiveness. Clinical Pharmacokinetics, 20, 1-24.

Yang, F. and Boissy, R.E. (1999). Effects of 4-tertiary butylphenol on the tyrosinase activity in human melanocytes. Pigment Cell Research, 12, 237-245.

Ziegler, V.E., Clayton, P.J. and Biggs, J.T. (1977). A comparison study of amytriptyline and nortriptyline with plasma levels. Archives of General Psychiatry, 34, 607-612.

Dark Matters - Dark Secrets **ISBN 1-884897-02-9** **$15.00 USD**

ABOUT THE BOOK

Dark Matters - Dark Secrets is the second book on the topic of melanin written by T. Owens Moore. As a continuing exploration into melanin research, Moore divides this book into two parts. In Part One (Dark Matters), the focus is on the role of melanin outside of skin pigmentation. Essentially, DARK DOES MATTER as a critical factor for the maintenance of life. In Part Two (Dark Secrets), a biopsychosocial approach is presented to discuss drug addiction and how the drug binding capabilities of melanin can make a person more susceptible to the effects of some drugs.

This book will be valuable to any reader interested in health and nutrition. The reader will obtain a unique outlook on the human body and learn new concepts related to the most complex entity in the universe, the brain. The emphasis is placed on how the pigment melanin found in dark skin and the melinated centers of the body are essential for proper physiological functioning. Astrophysicists use dark matter to describe the intriguing material in the external universe, and this brain scientist uses the term dark matter to describe the neuromelanin in the brain of the internal universe (the human body).

ABOUT THE AUTHOR

T. Owens Moore, Ph.D. is an Associate Professor of Psychology at Clark Atlanta University. For the past ten years, he has studied the neural and hormonal mechanisms that modulate behavior. He has published numerous scientific articles pertaining to the brain, and he is the author of *The Science of Melanin: Dispelling the Myths*. He is a well known educator in the Atlanta University Center. He has taught at Morehouse College and he is a member of the Neuroscience Institute, Morehouse School of Medicine.

To order **Dark Matters-Dark Secrets**, please fill out the order form below and send a check made payable to:

T. Owens Moore
Zamani Press
P.O. Box 667
Redan, GA 30074 (Allow 7-10 days for delivery)

Visit our website at www.zamanipress.com or fax orders to (770) 879-0275. Book stores and distributors can fax orders for special discounted rates.

ORDER FORM

Item	Quantity		Cost
Dark Matters-Dark Secrets $15.00		Subtotal=	
The Science of Melanin $15.00		GA Residents add 7% sales tax=	
		Shipping and Handling= ($3.50 for first book and $1.00 for each additional book)	
		Total Due=	